YOU'RE
TOO OLD
TO DIE YOUNG

YOU'RE
TOO OLD
TO DIE YOUNG

A Wake-Up Call for the
Male Baby Boomer on
How to Age with Dignity

DAN ZEMAN

www.DanielZeman.com
Scottsdale, Arizona

Patient privacy: With medical privacy laws, which I deeply respect, and my oath as a healthcare provider to maintain privacy, patient names, facts, and details have been changed, of course, to mask identities.

Medical disclaimer: The information contained in this book is not intended as a substitute for the advice and/or medical care of the reader's physician, nor are they meant to discourage or dissuade the reader from seeking the advice of his or her physician. If the reader has any questions concerning the information presented in this book, or its application to his or her particular medical profile, he or she should consult his or her physician. Neither the author nor the publisher shall be liable or responsible for any loss or damage allegedly arising as a consequence of the reader's use or application of any information or suggestions in this book.

www.danielzeman.com

Library of Congress Cataloging-in-Publication Data on file with the Publisher

Hardcover: 978-0-9600619-1-4

Paperback: 978-0-9600619-2-1

Mobi: 978-0-9600619-3-8

EPUB: 978-0-9600619-4-5

Audiobook: 978-0-9600619-5-2

LCCN: 2018914040

Printed in the United States of America

10 9 8 7 6 5 4 3

To the Greatest Generation, who delivered the baby boomers
into a time of great prosperity, ensuring them a longer
life-span and the freedom to make personal choices.

CONTENTS

FOREWORD

Every professional athlete realizes they will never defeat age and that someday each of us will be forced to retire. The biggest difference in retiring from sports is the age at which we are forced to retire. You begin to notice drop-offs in performance starting at age thirty, and by age thirty-five you find yourself unable to maintain those high-end levels of exertion that you did in your late twenties. If you add in the effect of injuries or accidents, the drop-off in performance becomes more frustrating.

As a former professional cyclist, I am proud of all my accomplishments—most notably, three Tour de France victories, 1989 World Championship, Jesse Owens Award, and Hall of Fame recognition. However, since I accomplished these before I retired, these are really only a piece of my life's legacy. Every athlete realizes his everyday life decisions do not stop when he retires from competition.

Dan Zeman, in this book, challenges every longer-living male baby boomer that his life's legacy is not written once they retire from an occupation. We all must realize that living longer provides us the unique opportunity to add, edit, or improve upon our life's legacy.

I met Dan in 1988 and quickly realized he was capable of performing the same level of cycling-specific metabolic (VO2) testing that I was getting in Europe. Dan had a VeloDyne, which allowed me to use my own road bike for all testing, and he used an analyzer that had to be calibrated against known gases. He knew the best testing protocols for professional endurance athletes.

Bottom line—he made my testing data reproducible, reliable, and valid.

I had injuries on and off the bike; the most severe was a gunshot accident. Dan was also very helpful as we tried to rule out the effect of the lead pellets in my body, my mitochondria changes, and my previous injuries, as well as accepting the fact that the level of performance needed to win the major cycling tour events had changed due to the influence of performance-enhancing drugs.

When you read this book, you will understand the impact medical advances will have on your longevity—which also means you, like me, have much longer retirement periods than any other generation in history. The years 2030 to 2050 will either be a time of great joy or sadness for an enormous chunk of retired Americans. The aging, retired male baby boomer needs to find something that will allow him to stay engaged.

I have been fortunate to have watched three men show me that the key to retirement at any age is to find something that keeps you engaged: my father (Bob), my wife's father (David), and Don (our longtime handyman) found reasons to remain active.

When I first retired, I booked speaking engagements where people wanted to hear my story about being the first American to win the Tour de France. One of the first was a talk Dan Zeman and I gave in Kalispell, Montana, at the Summit Medical Fitness Center. The audience was friendly and inquisitive about why I chose cycling, the value of setting goals, and a reminder that hard work does pay off. Unfortunately, later my talks became much more divisive as people struggled to admit cycling had a serious drug problem.

The great step for me and my family was getting involved in charities. The first was called "The Vietnam Challenge," which allowed US Vietnam Veterans, along with North and South Vietnamese Veterans, to ride bikes (traditional or hand cycles) across Vietnam. It proved to be a time of great healing, and we were grateful to be associated with the event.

Next, my wife and I helped create a charity called "1in6" for sexually abused children. Both of these charity events are great examples of finding something you are passionate about, and I encourage every aging male baby boomer to get involved with a charity as they plan their retirement.

My biggest positive take away from Dan's book is his desire to challenge the aging male baby boomer to understand their legacy.

Ironically, history will define us as players on an athletic team that either spent the last twenty-five years of their career complaining about getting old, or choosing to be a positive influence on the next generation who is waiting to get into the game.

Enjoy the book, as it will help you find more tailwinds than headwinds in your life's daily rides. It will also encourage you to find someone with whom you can share the beautiful views along the way.

Greg LeMond
Three-time Tour de France champion

INTRODUCTION

The year was 1946. A brand-new generation of babies was born in record numbers in America. Like me, you are probably one of them. Our generation would continue to grow until it reached 76 million faces and we became known as the baby boomers. As we began to age, each baby boomer remained uniquely motivated, yet still shared a common philosophy that each was going to stay forever young.

Today the stark reality for all baby boomers is we are no longer young. The first wave of boomers already kicked down the door marked age seventy; the second wave is turning sixty-five in record numbers of ten thousand per day; and the final wave will soon remember the number fifty-five as a speed limit they used to drive.

As a proud, grateful, and retrospective male baby boomer myself, I think our generation found its optimism, compassion, and sense of purpose from key milestone events like watching an American walk on the moon, witnessing the assassination of President Kennedy, and standing up against the Vietnam War or fighting in it. These and many other legendary milestone events provided the backdrop that quickly became the lyrics for the songs of our lives in the 1960s and 1970s.

Looking back, you could say it was easy being a baby boomer when 76 million of us were between the ages of twelve and thirty, but our enjoyment will drastically change when we are between the ages of seventy-two and ninety. Keep in mind, you can't hold back the sands of time.

As I see it, our generation's unique burden with the aging process is caused by our historic numbers as we will eventually total 19 million boomers over the age of eighty-five, and I intend to be in that group. Additionally, our rapidly deteriorating health status will mean America will have an unprecedented number of elderly citizens who will all need some degree of mandatory daily medical care, and, worse, the majority will eventually need 24/7 long-term assisted living care and housing. That's the group I don't intend to be in.

Even more troubling is our nonchalant belief that future generations will cheerfully accept the mental, physical, and financial costs associated with our poor health status, including diabetes, Alzheimer's, Parkinson's, cancers, strokes, obesity, heart disease, and depression.

The good news for every male boomer: the majority of us will not die young. That's also the bad news.

The good news for every male boomer: the majority of us will not die young. That's also the bad news. For those who want a more detailed glimpse of living longer, ask a fellow baby boomer who is currently dealing with an aging parent. He will either share happy stories of spending quality time together creating memories with grandchildren, or share painful stories about being forced to make decisions about his parents' driving, meal preparation, mobility, finances, housing, long-term medical care, and finally their end-of-life choices.

Keep in mind, knowing what's in your control and what's not in your control will help you make smarter and more realistic choices about how well you age. I wrote this book for my fellow male baby boomers (and for those who love them). After spending thirty-five years working inside the health, fitness, and sports medicine arenas as an exercise physiologist, performing thousands of exercise tests and designing exercise programs for individuals ranging from cardiac rehab patients to world-class professional athletes, I have made three simple observations.

1. **If you want to be a world-class professional athlete, then choose your parents very carefully.** It is clear to me that genetics plays the most significant role with regard to an athlete's ability to set a world record, because his genes determine his initial level of fitness, his ability to respond to intense training, and ultimately his maximal physical capabilities. Look at the growing list of professional athletes who are admitting to taking performance-enhancing drugs. In essence, most realize they are genetically inferior to other world-class athletes who naturally perform at a high level.

   The takeaway message for you is to set realistic fitness goals and maintain an exercise program that allows you to live out your life with the greatest quality of life. Do not continue to waste additional minutes, days, and eventually years of your life performing lengthy, single-focused, exhaustive exercise routines that only increase your risk of getting injured and cause additional physical and emotional fatigue. Your personal time is your most valuable asset. The amount of time you spend exercising needs to be viewed under the same microscope as any of your other assets such as your finances. Will you get a legitimate and justifiable return on your investment?

2. **If you want to live a long life, then choose when your parents were born.** I'm amazed at the number of male boomers who tell me about a medical procedure that saved their lives. Inevitably that revelation is followed by, "I wish that procedure had been available to my father, because the absence of it caused his death." The simple fact is, over the last one hundred years, the number of life-saving advances, robotic surgical procedures, and computerized medical devices continue to exceed

everyone's wildest imaginations. These advances are so profound that the average life expectancy has increased by almost thirty years.

As an exercise physiologist, I would like to believe today's exercise message is a key contributor to our increased life-span, but the simple truth is that medical advances have increased our life expectancy by both removing the major causes of premature death and inventing new treatments and procedures that drastically improve the chances of surviving conditions once deemed fatal.

The bottom line is that we are living longer because our generation's timeline allowed us to survive deadly childhood infections through access to newly developed, life-saving vaccinations. Our timeline also ensured we were born into a medical world that had just created both insulin and penicillin. And physical activity was just part of our daily lives in playgrounds and parks, and the efforts were applauded by the President's Council on Physical Fitness and Sports.

As young adults, we were the first generation to hear the widespread public health messages about the dangers of smoking cigarettes and the need for preventive medical screenings for cancer, heart disease, and stroke. We were born at the right time in the right place, which means we will live a long time.

3. **If you want to live independently and remain highly mentally, physically, and socially functional, then choose to do what your parents always told you to do.** Mom was right when she said "nothing good happens after midnight," and like it or not, Dad really did know

that "early to bed, early to rise, makes a man healthy, wealthy, and wise."

However, the simplicity of the observation gets more complicated for those of us who are currently struggling with an ongoing, troublesome medical condition. We need to rethink our current everyday lifestyle choices and realize we can no longer rationalize any destructive lifestyle habit. We need to adopt a healthier lifestyle— mentally, physically, and socially—as that will be the best predictor of our remaining quality of life.

Equally important is that every male boomer needs to understand that aging, all by itself, will force us to choose from an ever-changing list of good and bad choices. In other words, as we move through our six- ties, seventies, eighties, and nineties, we may have to adjust our sleep, the number of calories we consume, the types of physical activity we do, and the way we stimulate our brains. We are now aging baby boomers with a new list of health concerns. Whatever program or routine that worked for us in our twenties and thirties is no longer relevant.

The simplest way for us to comprehend our body's negative response to the aging process is to compare it to the positive responses of our youth. As teenagers, it was easy to accept that we could eat more calories, get by with less sleep, and still grow taller and stronger. In other words, youth is a time when your body naturally grew more cells every single day, while you remained relatively idle. Conversely, aging is a time when your body begins to struggle replacing or repairing those same cells. In this case, the going up was a lot more fun than the going down.

WE'RE NOT OVER THE HILL—YET

Today's aging boomer has literally become the group that was once classified as "over the hill." The major difference is how much longer you will spend going down that hill due to your longer life expectancy. Understand that the changes you begin to make today will drastically change how quickly you will go down that hill and how long you might lie motionless at the bottom of it. Let's hope not long at all—or ever.

In other words, the new perspective of every aging boomer should be to avoid being the person who was invited to a party but, in the end, everyone wished hadn't stayed so long.

My hope for this book is to remind the longer living male boomer that history will not remember how passionately we lived out our youth nor will it praise the lengthy list of creative accomplishments by a select few. Instead, it will wait to see how our entire generation chose to deal with the negative effects of an extended aging process that was forced upon all of us due to being part of America's longest-living generation.

Today's high-tech push-button world of automation all by itself has consequences. The cumulative effect of computerized technology has drastically reduced the number of our normal, simple everyday tasks to the point where physical inactivity has now become one of our biggest health concerns. The human body begins to atrophy when it is not actively engaged physically, mentally, and emotionally. In this case, the choice is not whether we choose to live in a high-tech computerized world; rather, it is our ability to choose how many minutes we spend being *motionless* in this high-tech world. This decision is one we make every day.

Thirty-five years ago, it was easy for me to promote the accepted medical position that structured exercise only needed to be performed three days a week. At that time, numerous studies showed people who exercised for thirty minutes, three days per week for a period of six to nine weeks could expect to burn off about 250 calories per bout of exercise. More importantly, they were able to decrease their percentage of body fat, increase their level of fitness, enhance mood states, and improve blood lipid levels.

My concern now is wondering if exercising for thirty minutes only three days per week is enough of an effort when we are living in a more automated and technologically advanced world. It is easy to forget that those early test subjects still lifted and lowered their garage doors, pushed their lawn mowers, got up off the couch to change the TV station, and walked to the mailbox every day of the week.

Failing to recognize that we no longer perform these simple daily tasks is significant, because each task contributed to the cumulative number of calories burned over the duration of the research studies. In other words, would those same exercise programs have the same positive health outcomes if the test subjects spent the majority of their day sitting in front of a computer screen, in a cubicle on the phone, or on the couch watching television?

The baby boomers are not the first generation to have benefited from milestone advances in technology. Early technological inventions such as electricity, the light bulb, the airplane, and the automobile were warmly welcomed and, to this day, continue to provide economic growth, as well as improve transportation and safety for every American.

Unfortunately, the same cannot be said for today's technological advances. While each can still be classified as milestones, the main focus is on improving push-button personal convenience and encouraging motionless mental entertainment, which means each new device has a physiological and psychological downside. Video games are a case in point.

Every aging boomer also needs to realize the role that today's automated technology has on decreasing his levels of muscle strength, balance, and flexibility, as well as his levels

Current research makes it easy to say that today's boomer burns off 400 to 500 fewer calories each day due to labor-saving devices.

of mental and physical attentiveness. Current research makes it easy to say that today's boomer burns off 400 to 500 fewer calories each day due to labor-saving devices. In other words, today's technological advances should really be considered as taking one small step forward for convenience but two giant steps backward for achieving a high quality of life.

The simple fact that having a poor quality of life is not because we stopped exercising for thirty minutes three days/week, but rather because we stopped being physically active during the majority of the week. Ironically, the proof of this connection is much more profoundly explained by asking any male boomer why there are so many more obese children compared to his generation.

My secondary hope for every baby boomer (man and woman) who reads this book is that we will begin to realize that history ultimately defines each generation by what it did for future generations. Our Greatest Generation parents made the world safer for us. In so doing, we are free to make choices, even poor health choices. Stated more bluntly, it will never be illegal to be unhealthy in the United States.

However, the converging timelines surrounding the baby boom generation (large population, longer life spans, life-prolonging medications, automated lifestyles) has made the decision to choose to be unhealthy more relevant because of its significant financial consequences. This is a debt that someone will eventually have to pay.

WHO LIVES, WHO DIES, WHO PAYS?

I believe the decision to take responsibility for making better health choices can be motivated by some profound perspectives. Consider the following.

- **National Perspective.** President John F. Kennedy in his 1961 inaugural address challenged us to "ask not what your country can do for you but what you can do for your country." My interpretation of his speech was that he encouraged people to get up from the couch and become actively involved in improving America. Instead, if we choose to accept our declining health habits, we would force our country (our kids) to introduce new automobile driving regulations, build and maintain hundreds of new assisted living care centers, as well as willingly absorb the monumental long-term healthcare costs from 30 million slow-reacting, uninspired, mentally diminished yet longer-living aging baby boomers.

- **Generational Perspective.** If the majority of aging male baby boomers are able to stay productive, it would rewrite how America has historically viewed the elderly. They would be seen as role models and not as a debt to our culture. We should attempt to be the first generation that learns how to age gracefully by accepting the natural decline in human function, yet still choosing to make positive contributions to society.

- **Personal Perspective.** By graciously accepting the bonus gift of an additional thirty years of life that is unique to our generation, now is the time to grasp onto this gift and get involved in those social issues you always promised yourself you would—if you only had the time.

MY PROMISE TO YOU

In this book, I bring my decades of experience working with the fit, the unfit, the willing, and the unwilling. I combine those experiences with the ongoing medical research that targets the negative effects that the aging process has on men.

I'll give you my best advice and strategies for action so your next thirty years can be filled with enjoyment and memories, not pain and suffering.

In the following chapters, we will

- Redefine the word exercise and realize it is no longer about being considered "fit" or "unfit." The new definition is to consider yourself as being "active" or "inactive."

- Follow the example of previous generations who were able to remain active throughout their lives because they had a secret ingredient.

- Work hand-in-hand with medical advancements that will keep you alive, but accept that having a life is up to you.

- Understand that today's push-button, automated, voice-activated technology has removed Darwin's theory of "Survival of the Fittest" and replaced it with "Survival by Siri."

- Encourage you to make better lifestyle choices. My goal is to minimize the risk of being injured or developing a lifestyle-related disease and save out-of-pocket health-care dollars. I call my list a healthier dirty dozen, and like Lee Marvin's gritty role in the movie by the same name, my dirty dozen may not change your mortality but will surely change your outlook on your life.

- Create a home program that includes flexibility, mobility, and agility movements that will allow you to live independently. The ability to keep all of these levels intact will be the difference between being "able" or "unable" to maintain what I call your nobility.

- Agree that investing time doing any type of physical activity has to provide a legitimate return on investment. The goal of having a healthy body allows you to endure more minutes doing things that you are passionate about, such as helping others.

The book also has an interactive website (www.danielzeman.com) that will encourage you to share, track, compare, motivate, and enjoy changing your daily lifestyle habits. You'll find videos and podcasts geared toward improving your quality of life. So find a comfortable chair, put on a pair of reading glasses, and enjoy learning how to prepare yourself to live longer, healthier, and happier than any other generation in history.

1

WAKE-UP CALLS— MINE AND YOURS

I had just finished teaching my first phase 3 cardiac rehabilitation exercise program. The program lasted six weeks and met on Tuesday and Thursday evenings in the lower level of St. Mary's Hospital in Minneapolis, Minnesota. The group included men and women between the ages of fifty and sixty-five, with different levels of fitness, education, social status, and household incomes. The only thing they all had in common was the medical diagnosis of having had a heart attack—and that they had survived.

I designed the entire cardiac rehab program and the theme of the room where it was going to be held. The class started with a five-minute group warm-up period, followed by twenty minutes of individualized heart rate training, and ended with a ten-minute cool-down that allowed for stretching and relaxation. I also included a ten-minute social gathering that encouraged participants to share their personal stories.

I was confident about the exercise physiology science part of my cardiac rehab program, but I knew I needed to consider all the other components if I really wanted the program to be successful. This included decisions about the overall theme and design of the exercise area, best time of day to meet, which pieces of exercise equipment to include, how many weeks of training to prescribe, and the optimal size of the group.

The good news was that my program seemed to be a hit with the cardiac patients. Most of them had big smiles and consistent attendance. I was satisfied with the success, but I wanted to design an even better program. So I handed out a questionnaire about their likes and dislikes and anxiously awaited the results.

The entire group's number-one like of my meticulously designed exercise program to assure their long-term survival after a life-threatening medical emergency was the plate of cookies I served during the social gathering. The number-two like was the cool-down period where they were able to lie down and listen to music. Needless to say, those responses were not what I had expected, but, nevertheless, those were their answers and my first wake-up call.

Thirty-five years have passed since that painful experience, but I still think of the insight it provided me. I learned that I needed to change my way of thinking. I had always thought the hardest part of teaching exercise was designing the perfect individualized exercise program. It turned out that's the easy part. The hardest part is teaching people to like exercise.

EXERCISE AS MEDICINE

I've always felt lucky to have been influenced by a number of outstanding individuals. The most significant is the physician who first believed in me, Dr. Herb Schoening.

The year was 1984. I had just finished my graduate degree in exercise physiology, and I found myself staring across the interview table at Dr. Schoening, an amazing physician with an impressive, innovative résumé—primarily because he promoted the use of exercise as treatment for a variety of diseases. He started incorporating exercise into his patients' rehabilitation programs early on in his medical practice before it became an accepted treatment.

Initially, he was involved at the Sister Kenny Institute in Minneapolis where he began using exercise as a treatment modality to improve the lives of polio patients. I remember Dr. Schoening telling me that although exercise was beneficial to polio patients, it was also possible for them to do too much exercise and actually make their symptoms worse. In other words, each patient had to exercise at an intensity level that was appropriate for their own ability or level of fitness.

This realization forced the medical research world to develop tests that could accurately measure each individual's level of fitness. These new tests allowed Dr. Schoening to see if another clinical population—that being the heart attack patient—would also benefit from the use of exercise as part of their rehabilitation program.

Keep in mind, in those days, the most common treatment for people who had a heart attack was up to a month of complete bed rest. Dr. Schoening told me he felt compelled to at least try something different for these patients because the majority of them died in that same bed.

The exciting news for me was that he offered me my first real job. I was confident that with his guidance, I was going to be able to persuade cardiac patients to exercise—and they were going to keep exercising.

The hidden bonus for me was that the hospital environment would also allow me access to patients with diabetes. At that time, the approach for treating diabetes was just beginning to include structured exercise programs. The research showed that exercise increased blood flow to the extremities, helped regulate blood sugar and insulin levels, reduced blood pressure, and was helpful to those diabetics who struggled to maintain an ideal body weight—all excellent outcomes to control diabetes and its miserable side effects.

The hospital programs were also expanding from a one-to-one patient-to-physician approach to a more inclusive medical team and family approach. The medical team included an endocrinologist, registered dietician, registered nurse, clergyman, and an exercise physiologist (that would be me). The reason for including the family was to identify a designated caregiver who would help buy groceries, encourage daily exercise, and supervise insulin injections.

Unfortunately, what took me six weeks of group training to find out about the cardiac patients' dislike for exercise only took one day to realize about the diabetic patient.

My first diabetic patient was a fifty-year-old sedentary man whose name is long forgotten, but I will call him John. I remember listening as medical team members discussed John's medical history and how his health had deteriorated to such a point where there was no alternative but to amputate his feet. I remember how quickly I had to walk by his room because I could not imagine how John would handle the devastatingly bad news.

What shocked me more was the possibility that John would rather have his feet amputated than start on a simple walking program. Certainly, there had to be something in John's personal past that was responsible for his initial and continued distaste for exercise. Maybe he had tried but felt embarrassed about his lack of athletic ability. Maybe he thought he really should start a walking program but was too busy. Maybe John believed he was too old to start exercising. Or maybe he just really, really hated gym class when he was in grade school.

Whatever John's reasons were for not wanting to exercise, it was clear to me that if I could not find the answer, I would not be able to help a majority of the diabetic patients.

I continued working at the hospital but struggled with the large number of patients who were unable or unwilling to take long-term control of their health habits. Most had a thirty-day window of success but then returned to their previous levels of smoking, overeating, or poor compliance in monitoring their blood sugar levels. They were able to convince themselves whatever put them in the hospital must not have been that big of a deal because they were still alive and happy to continue with their previous poor choices about their health. My second wake-up call.

EXERCISING FOR ALL THE WRONG REASONS

My next professional challenge led me to take a position in a revolutionary $17 million athletic club that included everything under one roof. This facility was the first of its kind and became the template for what is now called a four-season athletic facility. It had tennis and racquetball courts, every possible type of exercise equipment, basketball courts, meticulously clean locker rooms, and social programs. It also boasted an indoor fine-dining restaurant and an outdoor restaurant that even offered poolside meals.

It did not take me long to see a clear distinction between the hospital patient and the athletic club member. For the most part, the hospital patient was forced into an exercise program due to an illness or as an absolute life-saving necessity. The typical club member could not wait to return to their youthful habit of exercising. I was convinced that this basic motivational difference of actually wanting to exercise would allow me to be much more successful working with these members than I had been in the hospital setting.

From the very beginning, the typical athletic club member was excited and receptive to the concept of individualized fitness testing. They all found the data regarding their unique levels of cardiovascular fitness, body fat, flexibility, and muscular strength highly informative and wanted to compare their test scores to others in their age group.

It also became clear that the overwhelming majority of males were not content with just maintaining their levels of fitness;

they wanted to improve. Their single motivation was to be faster, stronger, and leaner than their buddies. It had taken me a few years, but I finally had found a group of people who actually wanted to exercise and also found the fitness testing data an essential tool for keeping them focused and motivated. Surely I had found my calling.

As time passed, it became clear that most of these men became compulsively driven to regain their previous youthful levels of fitness. Too frequently, that drive caused injuries, which forced them to give up and quit exercising altogether.

Even more disturbing to me was the number of men from thirty-five to fifty years old who informed me that the main reason for their daily two-hour workouts was to avoid the stress of trying to balance a wife and kids, home and job. I was also surprised at the number of twenty- to thirty-five-year-old men who were motivated to work out intensely for the sole purpose of being able to overindulge in food and alcohol without gaining weight. What? Wake-up call number three.

I remember feeling caught in the middle because I was unable to encourage the unhealthy hospital patient to achieve even a minimal level of fitness. Conversely, I seemed unable to get the healthy club member to feel comfortable enough with simply maintaining a moderate level of fitness for all the right reasons.

I must admit I did take a large degree of comfort when I heard that I was not the only health professional struggling with getting people to maintain an exercise program or to understand the magnitude of the benefits derived from exercise. As an example, a number of physicians struggled with the irony of their patients who asked about the benefits of exercise but never thought about quitting smoking.

Looking back now, I realize the importance of my time spent with the cardiac and diabetic patients inside the hospital, as well as with the members of the athletic club, because experiences with both groups were significant.

First, I had matured and improved my ability to be both assertive and compassionate when prescribing exercise programs. I learned to identify, understand, and motivate people across a greater age range. For example, I learned that the seniors (our Greatest Generation) wanted me to tell them only the basics about exercise. They had no interest in learning about all the confusing and boring exercise testing data. I think most were ready to quote the line from the movie *Gone with the Wind* and tell me, "Frankly, Dan, I don't give a damn."

I also found the aging baby boomer to be the easiest generation for me to identify with because I am one. That was all I needed to be viewed as credible—although it didn't hurt that I was able to recite the lyrics from the legendary songs of the 1960s and 1970s. If movies defined the Greatest Generation, music defined the baby boomers.

From a professional perspective, the passing of time allowed me access to a variety of new testing devices. I could test almost of any age, gender, height, weight, medical condition, or level of overall fitness. These new testing devices set the cornerstone for gathering longitudinal research that allowed the medical community to determine the amounts of exercise that were needed to remain healthy as we age. I was convinced that I would be able to persuade people to exercise, but this time it would be much easier because I had better testing equipment and more years of experience.

ENTER GREG LEMOND

I didn't have to wait long to test my theory. The first American and three-time winner of the Tour de France bicycle race, Greg LeMond, was getting ready to return to France in search of another victory. He asked me to regularly test and monitor his VO2 max (cardiovascular fitness) and percentage of body fat. I agreed, and we soon began a five-year testing program.

Every time I tested Greg, the scenario was always the same. He would bring in his road bike that he used in races, and we would mount it on a device that allowed me to create workloads similar to climbing the challenging mountains in Europe. The testing lab would have to be dead quiet, which was unique, because most people prefer to have motivational music playing in the background. World-class athletes are self-motivated. You never see them wearing headphones during a race. He would casually warm up and then tell me when he was ready to begin riding at an intensity that only a handful of people in the world could survive.

World-class athletes are self-motivated. You never see them wearing headphones during a race.

Next, Greg would look out over his handle bars and take one long blink. His eyes would go blank, and I would start methodically increasing the resistance. Throughout the test, we never spoke—primarily because those blank eyes made him appear to be strangely absent. The only sound was that of his rhythmic breathing patterns as they passed through a large mouthpiece that he wore so I could analyze the different levels of oxygen and carbon dioxide each time he methodically inhaled and exhaled. The only smell was that of burning rubber that was caused by the friction of his rear bike tire against the testing device's stainless-steel roller.

The test would always end the same way. He would simply look over at me and once again blink his eyes, and then he would suddenly return from wherever it was he went that allowed him to push those bike pedals so intensely.

To this day, I am still amazed how Greg was always able to push himself to pedal at a level of intensity equal to world-record power outputs inside my quiet testing lab. There were no large crowds screaming words of encouragement, the kind he was used to when climbing the action-packed mountain courses in Europe. It was just Greg, me, and my $50,000 metabolic analyzer in a quiet room in Minneapolis, Minnesota.

To those geeky exercisers who want to know the details, Greg's maximal cardiovascular fitness level was and still remains legendary at 6.2 liters/minute or 93 ml/kg/min. To this day, the number of athletes in the world who have ever recorded cardiovascular scores above 90 ml/kg/min remains less than a handful. What this means is that his heart, lungs, and skeletal muscles were able to deliver and consume oxygen at workloads that only a few others on the planet could tolerate. I also knew I would never again test or see this type of athlete in my lifetime.

I tested Greg as frequently as every two weeks. The goal was to compare his previous workload results to the most current. If his heart rate or the amount of carbon dioxide was lower than his previous test, then he was gaining a training effect. For Greg, this wasn't a time to rejoice; it was a time to increase the intensity of the next day's bike ride.

It had taken me six years, but I had finally found an individual who understood the benefits of a well-designed exercise program. The only major drawback of using Greg as an example of someone who could maintain consistent exercise adherence was that I found out that Greg really did not like exercise. For him, intense exercise was simply a means to an end—it was not a way of life. The frustration of losing a bicycling race was the single driving force behind Greg LeMond's lifelong commitment to exercise. My final wake-up call.

I now realize that Greg LeMond and Dr. Schoening allowed me to obtain an extremely rare perspective regarding the different levels of cardiovascular fitness across the widest possible range of subjects. With Dr. Schoening, I dealt with cardiac patients whose hearts were in such bad condition that they just stopped beating. With Greg, I saw a heart that was in such good condition that it was beyond comparison.

The most enlightening realization for me was that the actual heart muscle of any of the people I tested didn't know if it was riding a bike up a mountain in Europe, walking the dog, or sitting on the couch. Quite simply, how fast the human heart beats is left up to the heart's owner.

Once again it was clear that I was not in the exercise program design business. I was in the behavioral change business. I simply needed to find the reason or driving force that would persuade people to get up off the couch. Their hearts would do the rest.

THE EXERCISE MOVEMENT IS A COMPLETE FAILURE

As with my unplanned introduction to Greg LeMond, I soon crossed paths with another legendary man who shared with me a story about his ability to get a seventy-five-year-old man to start and maintain an exercise program. What made this man's perspective so valuable was that he had already acquired such an unrivaled reputation in the exercise world that he was simply known as Arnold.

Immediately after I mentioned that I was writing a book addressing the declining health and fitness levels of the baby boomers, Arnold Schwarzenegger shared with me a story regarding this older gentleman.

Arnold explained that although the man appeared to be healthy, he had begun to lose his ability to perform a variety of simple everyday tasks. Things such as opening jars, carrying luggage, and climbing stairs were becoming difficult for him; however, his most profound loss of strength was his struggle to stand up from a seated position without assistance. This loss of strength became particularly embarrassing for him because he was forced to search for restrooms where toilets were equipped with handrails.

Arnold explained to the man that if he began to perform some basic leg exercises, he would immediately notice a profound improvement in his leg strength and would no longer struggle to sit down and stand up. Arnold went on to tell me that he could not imagine how depressing it must have been for this man to believe that his continual loss of leg strength was just part of aging and that he would be forced to deal with this potentially embarrassing problem for the rest of his life.

I now believe for me to be successful at changing anyone's individual exercise habits, I need to recognize the degree to which an individual's generational timeline has influenced their belief or attitude toward the word *exercise*.

Some generations, as with my early cardiac and diabetic patients, believed exercise would be another short-lived cultural fad similar to the Hula Hoop of their time. This meant they were unable to view exercise with any degree of credibility and certainly not as a means of improving their ability to perform daily activities. The boomers were quick to blindly buy into the cosmetic marketing that promoted exercise as building "buns of steel" and "washboard abs." Younger generations chose to define exercise as something you needed to do only if you played youth or high school sports.

The good news was the medical world began to position exercise as medicine.

I also realized that in addition to my need to understand how each generation defined the word exercise, I needed to understand how the medical world and the fitness industry defined it.

The good news was the medical world began to position exercise as medicine. To them the lack of daily exercise had become so common and was linked to so many disease states that they were forced to create a new medical classification for their patients. They now not only define each patient by gender, age, height, and weight, they also refer to them as sedentary or physically active. It's right there in your medical records.

If the medical message was good news, the bad news was the message being promoted by the fitness industry began and ended with dollar signs. Late-night TV infomercials sold billions of dollars of exercise products, and programs promised thinner thighs, overnight weight loss, six-pack abs, and buns of steel—plus if you ordered whatever device or program being touted in the next three minutes, you could also get better sexual performance.

If you fast-forward to 2018 and take a look at the data regarding the current status of the exercise movement, you will understand why this chapter is a wake-up call, not only to me but to you, in so many ways.

- 75 percent of Americans fail to achieve the minimum standard of getting thirty minutes of daily exercise.

- 66 percent of Americans are considered overweight or clinically obese. The rates of obesity have risen exponentially over the last thirty years. Just look at photos of your grade school classmates. Nobody was obese, except for that one chubby kid in the back row, but we were told he had big bones.

- The medical community turned to the new line of pharmaceutical drugs geared at reducing the health risk associated with inactivity or obesity. They knew that Americans with high blood pressure, high cholesterol, type 2 diabetes, or coronary artery disease would rather take a pill than maintain an exercise program.

These statistics make it easy for me to admit that the exercise movement and its message of getting people to enjoy and maintain daily exercise has been a complete failure.

More importantly, as an aging male baby boomer, I am convinced it's time to get up and accept the wake-up call that details the failures of the exercise movement and to move on. None of us are getting any younger, and time is still our greatest yet depreciating asset.

As I see it, the importance of time and the philosophy of moving on need to be addressed by every aging male baby boomer (I call us the aging-MBBs) when he answers his annual birthday wake-up call. Milestone birthdays such as turning fifty, sixty, or seventy provide great motivation for men to refocus their use of personal time.

For those who prefer sports analogies, let's use the game of golf to understand that all of us are now playing the back nine holes of our lives. It is time to admit the reason most of us end up in the sand traps on the front nine is because of our lack of commitment to taking care of our golf swing. Likewise, for those who are currently in poor health, it is fair to say that most of us lacked a consistent commitment to healthy habits for the first fifty years of our lives. Every male baby boomer can make changes to his health and those will allow him to find great enjoyment playing the back nine holes of his life.

REDEFINE EXERCISE

My first suggestion to every aging-MBB is that you first redefine the word *exercise*. Start with the basic understanding that your heart and skeletal muscles have no idea what you are doing. They only know you are asking them to move. Understand that you no longer get additional style points for trendy exercise clothing or timely choreographed movement patterns. Nor should you care if the calories you burn come from mowing your yard, playing softball with your friends, or hiking for three days in search of the perfect campsite.

Exercise is nothing more than a conscious attempt to regain some levels of physical activity that you lost when you bought your first television remote control, push-button garage door opener, gas-powered lawn mower, or home computer.

My second suggestion is to forget about the amount of time and money you've spent trying to attain six-pack abs and beach-body biceps. Your new goal should be to achieve a level of fitness that allows you to comfortably move as many parts of your body as possible through the greatest range of motion until that day when you are standing over that final putt on the eighteenth hole of your life.

My original definition and belief about building exercise facilities was similar to the message found in the award-winning 1989 movie *Field of Dreams*—"build it and they will come." I really thought I would be able to convince Americans that this new concept of intense structured exercise would immediately become a national trend. I now realize there was a major flaw in my thinking.

In the movie, they didn't have to try to convince people they would like playing baseball. The game had already been invented, and each player already had fond memories of playing with friends and family members. The real message of the movie showed how much people missed playing baseball when they could no longer play it. Thus, my true mistake was neglecting to ask each person, "What is the activity you will miss when you can no longer do it?"

However, my biggest wake-up call was realizing everyday life in America had drastically changed. I can no longer view exercise as something that was invented with the hopes of increasing the quality and length of people's lives. Today's medical advances have made living longer all but a certainty. Today's technological community made our everyday lives so automated that we don't even have to get up off the couch to see who's at the front door. I now view being physically active as something that is mandatory because technology and medical advances have exceeded everybody's wildest imagination, and I address the intersection of those advances in the next chapter.

I can honestly say the biggest mistake that every aging-MBB can make is failing to consider the negative health consequences that are the result of living in today's automated, sedentary lifestyle. The simple truth is we will deteriorate—physically, mentally, and emotionally—more than we could have ever imagined because we have become so physically inactive.

My suggestion is to accept the fact that the majority of us will live into our nineties based solely on medical advances. Accept and appreciate today's push-button technology, but remember each new gadget reduces the number of calories we burn off each day by drastically reducing the number of minutes we're physically active. Most important, redefine the word *exercise* to mean any type of physical activity that involves movement, because increasing your level of daily physical activity will

The simple truth is we will deteriorate—physically, mentally, and emotionally—more than we could have ever imagined because we have become so physically inactive.

- Help prevent the loss of lean muscle mass and bone density that happens to every male starting at age forty,

- Help prevent the loss of brain function that is becoming a major concern for every aging male,

- Help maintain a positive outlook by ensuring you can still be an active, energetic, and productive aging male, and

- Improve your sense of balance, coordination, taste (yes, not a typo), and touch.

Ironically for me, perhaps the early cardiac rehab patients I encountered were correct in their likes and dislikes about my exercise program. They had simply forgotten just how good cookies really tasted!

2

SURVIVAL— NO LONGER OF THE FITTEST

In 1864 English biologist Herbert Spencer, not Charles Darwin, was the first to coin the phrase "survival of the fittest." After having read Darwin's *On the Origin of Species,* it seems Spencer thought his phrasing offered a better insight than Darwin's natural selection into the best predictor of long-term survival. The ability to predict survival rates is critical for today's aging male baby boomer, as he attempts to create a retirement budget based on the projected length of his life.

The ongoing debate concerning the lack of science behind a belief in survival of the fittest and whether it has any application to modern-day man continues to be challenged on many levels. My suggestion for every aging-MBB who is trying to predict his longevity is to ask himself one question: Why are so many baby boomers surviving longer than any other generation in the history of the United States?

I believe the simple answer is that we no longer live in the primitive civilization that was early America. It is easy to forget that there was a time not so long ago when survival was an every-day struggle of dodging deadly plagues and living in unsanitary bacteria-infested houses, and when not having access to any type of emergency medical care meant helplessly standing over and watching a loved one die a horrific death.

Today, Americans are literally cradled and coddled from birth to death between the hands of two highly advancing industrialized powerhouses. The first is modern medicine and its unimaginable life-saving advances, and the second is computerized technology and its high-speed, push-button, personalized, interactive world.

The goal of modern medicine has always been to create life-saving discoveries that will increase survival rates by removing the bad stuff that previously killed us. The medical advances of the first half of the twentieth century were so successful at introducing life-saving innovations that scientists were able to switch their focus to inventing life-extending advances.

Conversely, the goal of computerized technology is to create labor-saving products that reduce the amount of physical effort or exertion necessary to get work done. In other words, their primary goal is to improve our efficiency—which reduces our need to be physically fit.

The cumulative effect of these two industries has ensured our historic long-term survival rates.

Looking back, I believe the notion that our survival was tied to our level of fitness was, in part, due to the timeline of our birth. I was a child who grew up in the 1950s and 1960s, and it was easy for me to accept Hollywood's portrayal of survival of the fittest. Certainly, Superman's ability to save lives and leap tall buildings in a single bound was due to his level of fitness. Tarzan's ability to guarantee the survival of Jane among the flesh-eating lions was only possible because of his superior level of fitness.

Today's health clubs are another industry that chose to follow this proven marketing strategy of portraying peak fitness as the key to better health and long-term survival. One entertaining example is a thirty-second commercial entitled "Bears: Another Reason Y." This video portrays a group of millennials enjoying a hike in the woods. Suddenly, the loud sound of an angry growling bear prompts one of the hikers to yell "BEAR," which instantly sets the group into a frenzied race out of the woods.

The closing seconds show a smiling, confident woman leading the group out of the woods with conviction that she will survive. The video closes with painful screams of her least-fit fellow camper and the words: "Bears...another reason Y you should join." The goal of the video was to sell fitness memberships, not to educate the viewer on the difference between relative and absolute fitness levels.

I believe the best example of how Americans of all age groups have bought into the belief around needing to be the fittest is to compare the shift in New Year's resolutions. The earliest documentation of New Year's resolutions goes back to the 1930s when Americans were struggling through the Great Depression. A typical resolution then meant making a commitment to show gratitude for the things you had received—regardless of their cost—or to make a personal commitment to give of yourself to help others who were clearly less fortunate.

Today, one of the most common New Year's resolutions is to start an exercise program. Once again, the successful marketing of the notion of fitness convinced the majority of Americans that the key to finding health, happiness, and long-term survival meant improving their level of fitness. Fitness clubs and Ys filled up in January only to see dwindling numbers and broken resolutions by March.

So let me try to answer three questions:

1. Why are we surviving or living longer?

2. How fit do we have to be to survive?

3. What can we still learn from Charles Darwin's or Herbert Spencer's original beliefs?

A REVEALING TIMELINE OF ADVANCES IN HEALTH AND TECHNOLOGY

It is safe to say that if it were possible to gather the greatest medical minds of the last 500 years and challenge them to create new medical advances, none of them would or could have imagined the number and scope of life-saving and life-extending procedures that have been created since 1900. It is also safe to say that if it were possible to gather the greatest inventors of the last century and challenge them to create new labor-saving technologies, none of them—not even Edison or Ford—would or could have dreamed of the number and scope of touch-screen, push-button, interactive and robotic-enabled technologies that have been created since 1900.

The wake-up call for us is to appreciate the difference between how our grandparents survived and how our children will survive. To me, the answer is as simple as Survival by Sweat compared to Survival by Siri.

Let's consider a timeline that describes the unimaginable labor-saving devices that literally removed the sweat and the burden of maintaining a level of fitness in order to survive. At the same time, we'll examine the advances in medicine that prolonged lives—ours—and changed the face of survival in the jungle we know as life.

From 1900 to 1920, the medical discovery of different blood types opened the door for life-saving blood transfusions and today's blood banks. The American Red Cross says that every two seconds someone in the US needs blood, and approximately 41,000 donations are needed every day. Since blood can't be manufactured, it is still considered the gift of life. Blood literally and figuratively continues to save the lives of millions of people.

Another significant medical discovery documented in this time period was the spread of contagious diseases being linked to close living conditions, poor sanitation, and unsafe drinking water. The tragic story of Typhoid Mary provides the well-doc-umented case of a person's ability to consistently spread a deadly bacterial disease while remaining symptom-free. Her case rede-fined the notion of health and human hygiene and is the reason why handwashing has become customary in restrooms and the practice continues to save millions of lives.

The devastating 1918 Spanish Flu epidemic killed millions, and today's flu shots attest to the effectiveness of preventing another worldwide pandemic. But it was the emphasis on safe water and improved sanitation that led to sewer systems, which saved countless lives from deadly diarrhea—still an issue in developing countries.

Consider the period from 1920 to 1940 that included the Great Depression. You've heard people say a particular type of technology is the greatest invention since sliced bread. Yes, sliced bread became part of the American culture in the early 1920s and thus began the new goal of adding convenience to meal preparation. I have often said the main reason for the obesity problem in America is that food became easier to make, and we don't have to walk very far to get it. Radio became the place to gather around for news and entertainment, but soon became the place for sitting and eating too, which set the table for mindless eating in front of TVs in later decades.

Most still believe the automobile was one of the greatest technological inventions of this time period because it helped build the highways and interstates that allowed for interstate commerce, but it also removed the need to get all sweaty when hooking up the horse and buggy.

The discovery of penicillin still ranks as one of the top ten greatest advances in all of modern medicine. Prior to its arrival and use in the 1920s, the only option for people who developed skin infections from an accidental cut was to wait and see if they died. The first significant group of Americans who benefited from penicillin were the WWII soldiers. There was enough research to show that penicillin was effective in reducing the mortality rates that would certainly accompany the unpredictable number of cases of gangrene. Penicillin became an important part of the medical care for the D-Day landing in 1944.

Penicillin went on to become the most effective life-saving drug in the world by saving the lives of millions of people suffering from tuberculosis, gangrene, diphtheria, scarlet fever, and pneumonia. Today, penicillin is still saving lives by successfully treating bacterial infections of the ears, nose, and throat, as well as Lyme disease and pneumonia.

The second major discovery of this time period was insulin. Prior to the discovery of insulin in 1922, diabetes had always been recognized as a fatal disease, because the majority of diabetics died soon after diagnosis. The only medical treatment that showed promise was to put the diabetic patient on a very restricted diet of roughly 450 calories per day. This approach allowed the patient to survive a few more years, but most suffered with blindness, kidney failure, stroke, heart attack, and loss of limbs. Eventually all died of what could be termed as starvation. The discovery of insulin continues to save the lives of millions of diabetics.

The first significant group of Americans who benefited from penicillin were the WWII soldiers.

After WWII, historic medical discoveries and unimaginable technology and surgical procedures were introduced. Reports of polio were first documented in the late 1700s, but this infectious disease became more worrisome in the early 1900s and again in the 1950s. The discovery of the polio vaccine not only saved lives but also helped minimize the complications of the disease.

Childhood diseases came under control with discoveries of vaccines for measles, mumps, rubella, and pneumonia. No longer was pneumonia the "old man's friend"—the once common cause of death.

The other medically significant discovery of this time period was the successful use of vaccinations. Specifically, the mortality rate of infectious diseases such as diphtheria, pertussis, tetanus, and tuberculosis was drastically dropping.

The final major medical discovery of this time period was the potential benefit of using chemotherapy as a cancer treatment. This discovery was somewhat unintentional, as it was the result of observing the low white blood cell count in WWI and WWII soldiers who had been exposed to mustard gas. The first chemotherapy drug resulting from this research was appropriately named Mustine. Today millions of Americans use some form of chemotherapy in their battle to destroy deadly cancer cells because of this unintentional finding.

More calorie-saving technological advances were introduced into American homes in the 1940s and 1950s. The color TV with the newly designed remote control and the La-Z-Boy recliner introduced a new level of inactivity. Equally as impressive was the food and beverage industry's introduction of the Swanson TV dinner, tater tots, instant mashed potatoes, and the pop-top beer can. Kitchens began to look like the *Better Homes and Gardens* catalog with matching electric can openers, blenders, ovens, and toasters.

The days of burning calories while preparing meals were the next item on the menu with the introduction of the innovative Amana Radarange in the mid-1950s. The automatic garage door meant no more heavy lifting when leaving or returning to the comforts of a climate-controlled home. And the newly designed small gasoline engine was just beginning to change how we mowed our lawns and trimmed our hedges and trees.

With dreaded diseases eradicated through vaccines and sanitation, and chronic conditions under control with medication, the biggest shift in medical advances of this time period was driven by necessity, as heart disease now became the number-one cause of death in the US. The three biggest technological breakthroughs were the heart defibrillator, heart pacemaker, and the heart and lung machine. And medical history changed for good after the first kidney transplant in 1954.

By the 1960s and into the 1980s, home television programs were "brought to you in living color," and the list of cable channels—like our waist size—kept expanding. Every automobile switched to power steering, power windows, cruise controls, and automatic transmissions. The garages of most suburban homes rapidly became adorned with gas-powered lawn mowers, leaf blowers, hedge clippers, and snow blowers. We even created automated lawn sprinklers that allowed us to sit and watch the grass turn green. The roll-up garden hose was the next invention that allowed us to stand and power wash the cars in the driveway.

Outside of the home every store installed automatic doors, escalators, and elevators. Corporate America introduced the desk job, and people lined up to sit down. Even typing on an IBM Selectric gave way to lighter-touch computers with floppy disks.

From the 1960s to 1980s, there was significant success in the advancement of human organ transplants—not just kidneys, but hearts, livers, and pancreases, along with the invention of the first artificial heart. The success rate of these organ transplants was increased by the introduction of the first effective immunosuppressive drug—cyclosporine.

The introduction of computerized technology was also a significant medical advance, because it improved the clarity and accuracy of numerous life-threatening diagnoses. The invention of devices that use sound waves (ultrasound), magnetic resonance imaging (MRI), positron emission tomography (PET), or computerized axial tomography (CT-CAT) scans that provided both two- and three-dimensional viewing of the human body began to show up in emergency rooms, hospitals, and cancer centers.

During this time, lung cancer was officially linked to cigarette smoking, and the recommendation and acceptance of regular colon cancer screening became accepted. The ability to diagnose early-stage colon cancer or to completely avoid lung cancer has saved the lives of countless individuals.

In the last two decades of the twentieth century, the gas-powered labor-saving devices of the 1960s and 1970s became viewed as too heavy and bulky, so they were reinvented to be lighter and battery operated. The desire to stay home and watch movies became so popular that having a VCR and subsequent DVD player was viewed with the same mandatory perspective as having a flushing toilet or home telephone.

The office fax machine became the new "must have" labor-saving device to send documents, as it removed the need to walk to or stand in line at the post office. Also introduced was the single greatest new piece of interactive communication: the handheld cell phone. Its evolution continues to be amazing, as we all remember those early models as big and heavy as a brick and were convinced each new upgrade could never be improved upon. Now look how far we've come because I suspect your smartphone is at hand, especially if you're reading this book on your Kindle app.

By the last two decades of the twentieth century, the new medical focus was on improving heart surgery outcomes. New procedures included using a stent via angioplasty surgery or having open heart bypass surgery. These two distinct types of surgery have now become streamlined, and the majority of heart patients are out of bed and walking within twenty-four hours of surgery. The additional discovery of cholesterol-lowering drugs has allowed the arteries to remain open longer after surgery, as well as slowed the plaque buildup in those patients with a history of heart disease. The nationwide rollout of 911 emergency services also led to quicker arrivals to emergency rooms and more lives saved.

The increasing acceptance of routine cancer screening not only saved lives but began to remove the fear out of the diagnosis. Improvements in cancer screening procedures has also made them more convenient, which also led to a decrease in the death rates from lung, breast, prostate, and colon cancer starting in 1990.

Last year's model of anything is no longer cutting edge. Last year's touch-screen computer has already been replaced by voice-activated interaction. It is now possible to perform an ever-growing number of daily tasks while remaining completely seated without having to push a button. Technology's new push-button interactive computerized world has easily removed 500 calories each day from our previous daily caloric expenditures. (Just for reference, 500 calories is the rough equivalent of a four-mile run, every day of the week.)

> It is now possible to perform an ever-growing number of daily tasks while remaining completely seated without having to push a button.

Today, modern medicine is constantly being driven to create new cures, treatments, and procedures. The bottom line is to understand our long-term survival has evolved because modern medicine was able to provide treatments or cures to systematically eradicate the diseases that previously killed earlier generations. I categorize these medical advances as either life-saving or life-extending, but collectively they are the only reasons behind the increasing average life expectancy of every aging-MBB. These advances are so profound that the baby boomers should be renamed the "longer living" generation.

We need only look at the data from the CDC. A male baby boomer born in 1950 had an average life expectancy of 65.6 years. However, that same guy turned sixty-five in 2015 and now—thanks to those life-extending advances—is predicted to live another eighteen years. In other words, at his birth he was expected to live to the age of 65.6 years, but today his life expectancy has been extended to age 84.5 years.

THE LIFE-PROLONGING MARRIAGE
OF MEDICINE AND TECHNOLOGY

Looking back over the last hundred or so years of modern medical and computerized technological advances, it would be hard to decide which industry was the most impressive. Truth be told, the longer living, aging-MBB is the real winner, because the two industries are now in constant communication with ongoing updates. The new direction for increasing human survival rates involves a continually updating loop where improved testing technology improves the accuracy of a medical diagnosis, which then improves medical treatments, which in turn improves survival outcomes, leading back to improvement of testing technology.

The best example of this communication loop is the human genome project. Medicine knew that humans have twenty-three pairs of chromosomes, but it was the technology that allowed each chromosome to be further dissected to the point where each human is now defined by having 20,000 to 25,000 distinct genes. Most importantly, each gene is responsible for maintaining a specific level of homeostasis (in other words, maintaining a stable level among body systems) that ultimately determines life or death.

The ability to define a specific gene attributed to a specific medical condition allows for a new level of individualized treatment. The bottom line for the aging-MBB is that one day very soon our future survival will be determined by a computer's ability to read and interpret our unique human genetic code as objectively as today's architects read and alter a flawed architectural blueprint.

Until that day every male boomer only needs to understand the basics.

1. Your unplanned and increased survival rate is gifted to you by the coincidental timeline of your birth.

2. Your peak level of fitness (like your height) has been on a downhill slide since you turned thirty-five, and you no longer need to be fit to survive—modern medicine and technology are keeping you alive longer.

3. Your overall quality of life (like your muscularity) began to atrophy after you bought your first television remote control and the matching cozy sofa-style recliner.

Bob Dylan was correct in 1964 when he proclaimed to all of America how times were going to change. His prophetic lyrics are equally as relevant in 2018 but are now directed toward the longer-living baby boom generation. We are literally and figuratively changing the shape of America's age demographics. It always resembled the shape of a pyramid (a broad stable base of young energetic youth) but has lost its stability and became a new, more fragile shape (an abundance of frail elderly).

Today's CDC's age projections for the years 2040 to 2050 would certainly have Charles Darwin wondering how America is going to find space for 19 million elderly faces that evolution originally designed to have only 600,000 of us. Yes, the times really are changing.

As a young exercise physiologist, for me, it was easy to promote Darwin's belief in survival of the fittest. Certainly, the majority of Americans would not question the fitness message that "exercise will allow you to live longer." Unfortunately, the medical truth is every male baby boomer is gifted a longer life without having to perform strenuous and structured daily exercise at all. Americans have never shown the ability to consistently stick to a daily fitness or exercise program. Most realize adhering to a routine of taking prescription medications for high blood pressure, cholesterol levels, or a normal heart rhythm to be the simplest key to living a longer life.

Now, as a much older exercise physiologist, I still believe in the many benefits of exercising. The human body was designed to move, the heart to be engaged, and the brain to be challenged. Stated more bluntly, if the longer-living, aging-MBB is unable to motivate himself to remain physically, socially, and mentally active, then his bonus years will force him to contemplate the difference between being "alive" and being "kept alive."

The goal of maintaining a daily regime of physical activity is more important than simply living longer. Ironically, in the next chapter, I will use a generation of Americans who never heard mention of the word *exercise* to make my point.

3

FIND THE MISSING INGREDIENT IN EXERCISE

"The day the REA hooked up electricity to the farm" was the answer given me by my Great Uncle David when I asked him about the most important happening when he was a kid growing up on the family farm. My uncle was born in the early 1900s and grew up in the farm country of rural Minnesota. I am sure many other remarkable events happened in his lifetime, but getting electricity immediately came to his mind.

I couldn't imagine that I was talking to a guy who remembered when his house did not have electricity. Conversely, if I ask my nieces and nephews the same question, they would say Wi-Fi to power the iPhone or iPad was the highlight of their young lives. Ironically, my great uncle's generation and my nieces' and nephews' generation could both be classified as wireless—one lived in a house that had no electricity and thus no wires, and the others lived in houses where every piece of technology was wireless.

Regardless of your generational timeline, today's increasingly widespread acceptance from the ever-growing list of unimaginable technological advances will continue to impact all of us. Initially every new piece of technology was designed to improve job efficiency but now interactive touch-screen devices are literally at everybody's fingertips.

Like no other time in history, it is now easier and more fun to sit completely motionless on the couch and still be highly entertained. Unfortunately, research has also clearly shown that adopting a sedentary lifestyle increases the risk of heart disease, diabetes, high blood pressure, stroke, and obesity. These two opposing scenarios define my new daily challenge: How do I encourage someone to become more physically active when being completely sedentary is so much fun?

I am convinced the answer to why some people are able to maintain a daily program of regular physical activity—while others struggle to get up off the couch—is really a question of how and what we perceive to be fun. Once again, it was one of my elderly relatives who provided me with unique insights into whether being physically active was ever fun.

In the mid-1980s, I was proudly giving my seventy-five-year-old Grandpa Walker a tour of the Flagship Athletic Club in Eden Prairie, Minnesota. The Flagship had earned national recognition as a state-of-the-art fitness facility. I even waited until 6:00 p.m. so he could get a feel for the large number of members who stopped by the club to exercise after they finished work. I remember watching him as he stood gazing at the hundreds of members running, riding stationary bikes, and lifting weights.

I was expecting him to say, "Wow, it looks like these people are really having fun."

Instead he turned to me and asked, "Don't these people get too tired to exercise after working all day?"

My grandfather continued to stare in disbelief at the number of members who were endlessly stepping up and down on the Stairmaster but going nowhere and those who were lifting forty-pound weights but not carrying anything of significance anywhere. My guess is that he couldn't comprehend his fellow farmers going someplace after an exhausting day of field work so they could burn off calories without actually lifting something or going somewhere. To him, exercise had no legitimate purpose, and having the energy or desire to exercise was easy if all you did was sit on a comfortable chair all day.

The really good news for my grandparents' generation is they were able to reap the physiological and psychological benefits of daily physical activity without having to buy a membership to a fitness center. I tried to explain these bonus benefits of farming, but all they knew was that their hearts and bodies were completely fatigued at the end of each day, and their arms and legs ached.

We know that daily physical activity improves cardiovascular health, maintains muscle mass, and burns calories. It would be a mistake to think these training effects could only be reaped if my Grandpa Walker was on a treadmill, dressed in spandex inside an air-conditioned athletic club.

We also know that physical activity affects your brain. Most people say being active makes them feel better, which in turn allows them to tolerate stress. Medical research points to changes in endorphins (these are the feel-good chemicals in the brain released by activity) that are responsible for an individual's mood change and has clearly shown that maintaining even mild levels of physical activity are beneficial to those who are suffering from depression.

Most people say being active makes them feel better, which in turn allows them to tolerate stress.

This exercise and mood state connection most certainly played a role in how my grandparents' generation was able to remain physically active during the 1930s. Keep in mind that staying physically active during a time that has become known as the Great Depression had to be difficult. Ironically, today many individuals cite physical or emotional "stress" as the main reason why they are unable to find the motivation to perform any type of daily physical activity/exercise, when that very activity would boost their mood and lift them out of depression.

My grandfather's tour of the Flagship Athletic Club did not turn out the way I had planned. Looking back, the statistical nerd inside of me would have enjoyed gathering data on the lives of those hard-working family farmers:

- Would those family farmers—who already demonstrated a lifelong adherence to daily physical activity out of necessity—have found any fun spending thirty minutes, three days a week, walking indoors on a treadmill after a full day of farming, or would they have complained about being too tired?

- Would this nonstop, hard-working generation have allowed themselves to become completely sedentary by sitting on the couch watching TV or playing computerized games eight hours a day, if that type of technology had been invented? (Maybe nonstop physical activity was simply part of their generation's genetic code.)

Although I will never know the statistical answers to either of these two questions, I was able to get my Great Uncle David and my Grandpa Walker to share with me the amounts of daily physical activity that were forced upon them by simply being born in the early 1900s.

The wake-up call for both of my relatives came about 5:00 a.m. Time to put on a pair of bib overalls (no fleece-lined spandex for farmers) and walk outside to the cold, smelly barn. The first two hours included feeding the cattle and then filling buckets of milk one squirt at a time. Next it was off to breakfast, which of course included manually pumping a five-gallon bucket of fresh water and building a fire in the wood-burning stove (no microwaves, running water, or electric stoves in those days, and guess who split that wood and started that fire?).

After breakfast, it was back to the barn for another three hours of shoveling manure and carrying feed to the horses, pigs, and chickens. Chores also included any mandatory maintenance, as it was hard to call the local fix-it shop without a telephone. The rest of the day included five to six hours of field work, followed by a three-hour repeat of the animal chores in the evening. This seven-days-a-week routine became the norm for the first thirty-five years of their lives.

I was glad to hear the intensity of their everyday work efforts did eventually decrease as they—like all generations to follow—gladly welcomed technological advances that allowed them to get the same amount of work done but burn fewer calories per day.

The early research communities never tried to make a connection between technological advances and the number of calories burned, because nobody viewed increased work production as a having a downside. The connection didn't become apparent until the majority of the American workforce had switched to sedentary desk jobs and homes were filled with TV remotes. The rising rates of heart disease, high blood pressure, adult onset diabetes, and obesity—now that's the obvious downside.

Today, researchers at the Centers for Disease Control and Prevention and the American College of Sports Medicine are outspoken about the positive health benefits of regular physical activity. They define the recommended amounts of daily physical activity in terms of aerobic exercise (for heart and lungs) and strength training exercises (for muscles).

The recommended bouts of strength training call for a minimum of at least two days a week. The weight should be continuously lifted and lowered eight to twelve times or until the muscle becomes fatigued (in other words, you could not lift that barbell even one more time). Ideally the strength training program should involve the major muscle groups of the arms, chest, legs, and abdomen.

When my grandparents were farming, examples could have included a variety of daily activities, because every task involved some type of lifting and lowering. The simplest scenario would be the twice daily carrying of the twenty pounds of milk in a metal bucket produced by a single cow (not to mention the squeezing and pulling it took to get that milk in the bucket). It would be a mistake to assume the muscles of the arm obtained additional strength benefits from lifting chrome plated dumbbells in comparison to lifting a milk bucket.

Today's guidelines for the desired amount of aerobic activity encourages the typical American to set aside at least 150 minutes each week (could be thirty minutes, five days a week) for activities such as brisk walking. Once again, it would be foolish to assume that my Uncle David was unable to meet these guidelines when the only way to get from the house to the barn on those cold winter mornings involved a very fast-paced walk. And farming was a seven-day-a-week aerobic activity program.

I would have enjoyed designing a study comparing and contrasting the average and maximal daily heart rates of the active farmer with those of today's typical health club member. But knowing my Great Uncle David, it would have been a real struggle to encourage him to put on a heart rate chest strap on the way out to the barn at five in the morning.

The key takeaway regarding strength training and aerobic activity is that both of my relatives easily exceeded today's guidelines for the recommended amounts of physical activity—and they did it every day for the first fifty years of their lives.

Some of today's exercise gurus are quick to defend their clients' inability to consistently maintain a five day/week exercise program by stating "everyday adherence to physical activity was easier for their grandparent's generation, because physical activity was how they made a living," or even stating, "physical activity was a matter of life or death to that generation."

No question, our agrarian grandparents' livelihood depended on being physically active. I also freely admit the specificity of training and the peak intensity of their efforts were far less demanding than those of today's typical fitness club member, especially those who are training to run a marathon or competing in a body building contest. However, if you compare the total number of minutes of daily physical activity or the total number of calories burned, the earlier generations in bib overalls were vastly superior to today's spandex-clad fitness club member.

Life or death? If physical activity was a matter of life or death for the Greatest Generation, then being physically active is a matter of life before death for the baby boomers. This is an important distinction because boomers have a much longer average life expectancy than those of earlier generations.

If physical activity was a matter of life or death for the Greatest Generation, then being physically active is a matter of life before death for the baby boomers.

LOOKING FOR FUN IN ALL THE WRONG PLACES

You, my fellow male boomers, will be the first generation to live out the remaining years of your lives with the least amount of bone density, muscle mass, cardiovascular function, hand-eye coordination, physical balance, and quite possibly the highest levels of body fat. This is an important distinction because these greater physiological losses will mean even greater losses in daily mobility to the point where it will cause a drastic loss in the quality of your lives.

Exercise research has already shown that one of the reasons why most people choose not to exercise (become physically inactive) is they find it to be boring or "not fun." Today's sedentary aging male baby boomer believes structured exercise has a purpose; he has access to exercise equipment; he understands he will live well into his late eighties; yet he still will not put down the TV remote and get up off the couch. Sound like someone we all know?

Perhaps you are looking in the wrong place. Once again it was my elderly relatives who first pointed out that everyday farming was not fun, but being a farmer brought them great joy. In fact, I had never seen either of them laugh so effortlessly as they did when they told me stories about life together and the fun they had on the farm. It has taken me thirty-five years to understand that without some type of social interaction, long-term compliance to daily physical activity is impossible.

The best example I've experienced with aging-MBBs who were able to find the fun within an intensely structured exercise program was when a group of fifty-five-year-old physicians approached me with their idea of doing a group bike ride. They wanted to know if I would design a comprehensive bike training program that considered their age, heart function, relative level of fitness, leg strength, and busy work schedules. My problem was they didn't just choose any old casual friendly fun bike ride. They chose the 2,975-mile Race Across America (RAAM) ultramarathon bike ride that started in Oregon and ended in Florida—and they wanted to do it in less than eight days!

The biggest obstacle with this type of bike ride is it involves nonstop twenty-four-hour efforts. Creating a relay team of four riders was a requirement, which meant one of the four riders would always have to be pedaling until they reached Florida. Other racing obstacles included uncontrollable factors such as temperature, humidity, wind, altitude, and the elevation of climbs, making it impossible to predict the number of watts (workload) each cyclist would experience. Collectively, these obstacles could be minimized if each rider needed the same amount of time to rest and recover, but these four guys wanted to arrive at the finish line in Florida as a team in less than eight days.

My first thought was there had to be a small leak in the anesthesia tanks inside the surgical rooms. They believed their strong social connection would make riding across the United States in eight days an achievable goal—and they convinced me. They also told me they were planning on calling themselves Team Viagra. With a name like that, they planned on having fun.

We first scheduled a kick-off fitness testing day where each physician had his VO2 max, anaerobic threshold (AT), and percentage of body fat measured. Along with knowing their previous training schedules and current surgery schedules, these data allowed me to prescribe an individualized training program for each physician.

The challenge behind designing an intensely structured exercise program is that it requires a balance of making the efforts demanding enough to improve the subject's level of fitness yet still keep them mentally tolerable. Designing a training program for a nonstop 2,975-mile endurance ride had another caveat, because it also had to include multiple daily workouts at various times of the day. Although each physician continued to periodically ask for my professional training advice, they also became equally interested in how each teammate was staying motivated to keep up the demanding training schedules.

Initially, they shared helpful tips pertaining to the safest roads in and out of town or the best way to balance their work schedules. Equally important was their ability to humorously warn each other as to which foods not to eat before going on long rides (private restrooms aren't strategically placed along the roads), or which cycling shorts do not provide a sufficient amount of padding. However, the most important thing they realized was that their passion for finishing the ride kept them motivated to train as a team.

Ultimately, these four docs achieved their goal of riding from Portland, Oregon, to Gulf Breeze, Florida, in under eight days—plus ended up riding under the name Team Heart, which raised a significant amount of money for children battling heart disease. I ran into one of the physicians recently. He smiled as he remembered how much fun he had doing the RAAM ride. He didn't say, "Dan, those daily cycling workouts you designed were unbelievably challenging," instead saying, "Dan, I can't begin to tell you how much fun we all had." His ability to remember only the fun of doing the RAAM ride and forget about the necessary daily exercise program clearly underscores the importance of creating a social connection to ensure exercise adherence.

It works the same way for other aging-MBBs whose exercise programs are nothing more than the means to an end for a fun social event. I can think of several occasions: The time Chuck asked me about getting in shape so he could finish a 10k charity run with his athletic son, or the time that Jim said a bunch of his buddies wanted to take their sons on a weeklong hunting trip but he could barely walk a mile without getting tired, or the time that Ray asked about getting in shape for a group hiking and canoeing trip in the boundary waters of northern Minnesota. Once again, none of the guys later complained to me about the drudgery of their lengthy, intense training exercise program but began with the simple positive statement of "we had so much fun!"

One of the biggest mistakes today's structured fitness move-ment continues to make is trying to convince the male boomer that he will find fun doing structured exercise. In doing so the majority of these men ended up feeling they were mentally or physiologically flawed because no matter how hard they tried, they never found the fun.

Let me be the first to say to the overwhelming majority of those who believe they are fitness failures: You need to step back and develop a fresh perspective about structured exercise. In other words, it's time to move on.

RX FOR FUN

My recommendation for the majority of aging-MBBs is to stop viewing exercise as an intensely fatiguing, mandatory daily task, but instead view it as a way of maintaining a social connection among old friends. You should put down the TV remote and contact a friend, old college buddy, or family member with whom you share a cultural passion.

If you are passionate about nature, for example, then create an email challenge to see who can go outside and take the most colorful photos of regional wildlife. If your passion is music, architectural design, or wine, it will become apparent that the more physically active aging-MBB will have the most fun sending the most creative photos of himself standing in front of music concert halls, stone bridges, or sprawling vineyards. If your fellow boomers live nearby, then choose a local seasonal event that combines activity, education, and maybe a charitable contribution that everybody can rally around. If you can't agree on an event, you can simply start your own by doing seasonal yard work for those who are physically unable.

The key point is to realize the fun will not be found in the daily preparation, but with the smile that comes from the memory of completing the event. Most important, every aging-MBB needs to challenge himself to keep searching for passionate activities that allow him to find continued fun as he lives out the extra years of his generation's extended lives.

> **The key point is to realize the fun will not be found in the daily preparation, but with the smile that comes from the memory of completing the event.**

My belief is if we choose to redefine the term exercise, then the number of calories that can be burned, the distance that can be walked, or the amount of fun that can be shared among friends will make being physically active a means to an end.

My grandparents' generation did not find fun in working those long hours on the farm. They found fun in talking about farming with other farmers—you'll see them at nearby small-town diners and highway truck stops having coffee every morning. The physicians who rode across America did not find fun in training for the ride. They found fun in sharing their memories about the ride. The aging male baby boomers among us need to understand we won't always find fun in being physically active, but we will find unparalleled fun in sharing our life passions with others and remembering that our hearts don't know if we are wearing running shoes—but our hearts will know if we had fun.

4

RETIREMENT: SO NOW WHAT DO I DO?

Every aging-MBB needs to accept the fact that his increased life expectancy also means a longer period of retirement. Now that we know why we are living longer than any other generation, it's time for each of us 35 million aging boomers to ask and answer a more relevant question: "How much will each additional year of retirement cost?"

As I see it, the simplest answer is that it depends on how many of your final years you spend in an assisted living facility.

I am not the only one who believes everyone needs to answer this question. Dr. Atul Gawande does a fabulous job discussing the emotional topic of death in his best-selling book, *Being Mortal*. He also points out one of the biggest differences between today's elderly and those of earlier generations: the location of their death. He said, "As recently as 1945, most deaths occurred in the home. By 1980, just 17 percent did." Today, he said, "The experience of advanced aging and death has shifted to hospitals and nursing homes."

While I agree with Dr. Gawande's statement that the majority of aging-MBBs will eventually end up in a nursing home or an assisted living facility, I believe the following questions should provide the biggest wake-up call for every one of us.

1. Who makes the decisions as to when you can no longer live independently?

2. How do you minimize the number of years you might live inside an assisted living facility?

3. How many of your final months will you be totally dependent upon others for your daily care?

Once again, I prefer to keep things simple. The answer to all three of my questions can be found by looking at the preadmittance form to assisted living facilities. The intent of the form is to get a detailed understanding of the person's ability to perform tasks using the following four categories: personal care, physical mobility, personal housekeeping, and emotional status.

For example, each person is asked about their current ability to perform everyday tasks such as bathing, climbing stairs, doing laundry, managing finances, socialization skills, and the ability to follow instructions. Most people mistakenly believe they will be able to openly discuss their physical, emotional, or social abilities, but unfortunately, the questionnaire only allows for a single check mark. You either put a check mark in front of the word *able* or *unable*.

In essence, the net result from every decision you make about your physical, emotional, and social well-being is added up and instantly declared able or unable. You will not have the option of checking "sometimes" or "it depends." You can either get up out of bed and get dressed without help or you can't.

Initially, I found the questionnaire's simplistic approach quite harsh and judgmental. However, the truth is every one of us aging-MBBs has already began to notice some type of physical, emotional, and social red flags and has brushed them off as being insignificant or no big deal. For example, do you struggle to put on shoes and socks? Have difficulty looking over your shoulder when driving a car? Fumble with small buttons on shirts? Lack strength when carrying groceries? Can't keep your home clean? Lose your balance when walking up or down stairs? Sometimes don't want to talk to other people?

In other words, no aging-MBB can expect others to feel sympathetic to your situation, nor believe you just woke up one day without any warning and found yourself physically, emotionally, or socially "unable" to take care of yourself. But that is the final straw of deciding when you will be admitted into assisted living.

Another reason for educating ourselves about assisted living centers is based on the logistics of forcing 19 million baby boomers into assisted living centers given our country's challenges with designing and maintaining such facilities for other large segments of our population.

Starting in the late 1800s there was a belief that unwanted or orphaned children could be safely housed and properly educated in so-called state schools, but this proved to be a failure and all were eventually closed. A similar housing scenario was implemented to provide better medical care and safety for those once considered to be mentally or physically challenged, but those facilities also proved to be difficult to justify given their outcomes.

Most recently there has been a consistent demand for better housing and medical care for military veterans. This group has the big advantage of being political front-page news, yet America still struggles with meeting their needs.

The wake-up call for the aging-MBB is to understand that the challenge has never been identifying a segment of the population that needs 24/7 dependent care. Rather, it has always been the ability to provide dignified care—medical, emotional, and cognitive—at a justifiable financial cost.

I have always found that men really do not fear dying, as we all know that death is a certainty. The majority of male boomers understand they need to budget for assisted living, but their biggest fear is being totally dependent on others and having zero quality of life. Keep in mind, previous generations were able to avoid budgeting for assisted living facilities because most who retired at age sixty-five died shortly thereafter.

The baby boom generation needs to understand the flaw in the popular statement, "America is getting older." Worse, this statement is validated by the statistic proclaiming "every day in America 10,000 Americans turn 65 years of age." The obvious flaw is America is not getting older. The baby boom generation is getting older becuase they did NOT die young!

Modern medicine and technology have allowed the largest generation in history to reach sixty-five, and modern medicine's continual desire to introduce life-extending treatments will force every aging-MBB to recalculate the financial impact of a longer retirement period.

It's not about what you are going to do with those extra years, it's about how healthy you will be during those years and who will eventually pay for your care when your health declines and you can no longer care for yourself. We can learn from the professional athletes among us.

AGE AND ATHLETES—THE ONLY OPPONENT THEY COULD NOT BEAT

I have been fortunate to have worked with world-class athletes for many years and am still amazed at how these high-level athletes always respond so superiorly to the everyday athlete, even though they are doing the same training program.

My single takeaway from dealing with the best of the best is that each shares the common denominator of early-age athletic success. Each found it easier to bike, run, swim, throw, and jump significantly faster, longer, or farther than others of their age group. As they went through puberty, the slope of their physical improvement continued at a faster pace until they were forced to compete against older athletes. Each would also say that from age twenty to twenty-seven, their levels of sport-specific fitness (strength, quickness, agility, cardiovascular endurance, hand-eye coordination) continued to improve as long as they practiced each skill set.

Each athlete also expressed times during this period where his peak performance seemed surprisingly effortless, or that the speed of his performance just seemed to slow down as if time became elongated. They often stated they were just in a zone where they knew they would win.

However—and here's the lesson: Every professional athlete, will eventually have to check the box marked *unable*.

In their case the ability to outperform their competitors began to change as they approached age thirty. Most stated they needed more rest days to recover before they could compete again. But if they took too many days off, they would begin to notice a drop-off in their performance because of the prolonged inactivity.

Unfortunately, all of them eventually realized their days of setting world records or winning world championships were coming to an undeniable end.

Ironically, their brutal wake-up call was not realizing they were no longer the fittest; rather, it was accepting that they had not reached thirty-five years of age. In other words, each had to accept that aging was the only opponent they could not beat and their period of retirement was going to be a struggle.

I believe the world-record holder offers the following two insights to every aging-MBB as he attempts to plan for his retirement.

1. Every world-class athlete had to find something new to do after his retirement—knowing it will never match the same level of enjoyment or physical or emotional intensity.

2. Every world-class athlete initially viewed inactivity as rest but soon realized that his body began to atrophy when the number of days off became excessive.

NOW WHAT?

The thought of retirement for any pro athlete (and for the rest of us) has been on his mind since he started working those mandatory forty-hour work weeks. The only difference between the aging-MBB and the world-class athlete is when they start their retirements. The longer-living, aging-MBB has to decide what to do after about age sixty-five, while the world-class athlete needs to decide what he's going to do after age thirty-five.

Yet they both share a simple understanding and need to accept they may never experience the same physical and emotional level of personal satisfaction they once enjoyed in their completely separate career paths.

The potential mistake the aging-MBB can make is failing to see the connection between the athlete's inability to walk away from his passionate identity of being a world-class athlete to his own inability to walk away from his passionate identify found in being a police officer, business owner, factory worker, salesman, teacher, construction worker, physician, or mailman.

One of the fundamental hallmarks of the male baby boomer is his pride in what he accomplished outside of the home. The sense of pride he gathered from his accomplishments during his forty-year occupation became part of his identity, and the fear of losing that identity mirrors the fears of the world-class athlete. The timing of the loss just shifted from thirty-five to sixty-five.

The key for the longer-living male boomer is to look at retirement as another legitimate and productive phase of your life and not just a short-term ending to a life you already lived. You should not waste your opportunity to get back in the game of life.

THE INACTIVITY TRAP

Every world-class athlete realizes he simply responds better to the same stimulus or amount of exercise as his competitors. I now realize that his gifted response is actually a twofold phenomenon. It is easy to understand that he responds better because he can outperform his competitors. It's the second phenomenon that gets forgotten. Each world-class athlete also recovers faster from the same bout of exercise. This allows him to train with the same intensity the very next day.

I learned this from working with Greg LeMond. The Tour de France is a grueling, month-long professional bicycle race. The eventual winner is the cyclist who can get up every morning and continue to ride his bike, day after day, at world-class speeds but still outperforms the other cyclists who had the same amount of sleep. But as every young world-class athlete begins to age, regardless of his sport, he recognizes that an additional day of rest is the only way for better recovery from intense exercise.

Unfortunately, increasing the number of rest days or inactive days only causes him to atrophy to the point where his previous easy training efforts have now become more troublesome. In other words, he is still able to train intensely, but his level of performance just keeps decreasing.

He also realizes that the drop-off is not subjective because he lives in a measurable world where everything can be documented. His maximal heart rate drops, his race pace slows, his power output drops to the point where he is no longer capable of setting world records. Eventually each world-class athlete understands that his rest days begin to outnumber his training days. And while he is still considered to be among the fittest, he is no longer fit to compete at the world-class level and he must retire.

The key takeaway for every longer living, aging-MBB is to understand if he chooses to have prolonged days of inactivity, then he will notice a drop-off in his ability to perform daily tasks.

He literally will go from being able to perform a task to being unable. In essence, the quickest way to be forced to retire into a resting home is forgetting that resting is what put you there!

The great news for every aging-MBB is the ability to put a numerical value on any type of physical activity—that measure is not exclusive to the world-class athlete. Researchers began using the mathematical measurement of MET levels in the 1950s, which offers great insight for the longer living, and now retiring aging-MBB who is trying to stay out of assisted living facilities.

The acronym MET is used to describe the metabolic equivalent of a task. It is based on the science behind human metabolic rates. This mathematical calculation suggests that all humans are at 1 MET (metabolic equivalent task) when they are at rest. One MET is then used as a baseline multiplier when comparing different activities or daily tasks in relative terms.

For example, a particular activity with a 2 MET level is one that requires two times the amount of energy that is expended at rest. Likewise, a 3 MET activity requires three times the amount of energy that is expended at rest, and so forth. Most importantly, this calculation also allows the comparison between every daily task and exercising on any piece of equipment (such as a stationary bike, treadmill, or stepper).

...understand if he chooses to have prolonged days of inactivity, then he will notice a drop-off in his ability to perform daily tasks.

The ability to cross match levels of effort was the early foundation of hospital-based cardiac rehab programs. The goal was to ensure a patient's safe return to work after open heart surgery. The typical scenario involves a cardiac patient who wants to return to a physical job that requires an exertion equal to 7 METs. He is able to mimic the 7 MET level of exertion on a stationary bike inside the safety of the hospital while simultaneously monitoring his heart via an EKG. If he is "unable" to show competence or the ability to exert 7 METs on the stationary bike, then he is "unable" to safely return to his physically demanding job.

Today's broad-based MET charts include an extensive list of specific tasks but can be generically categorized in terms of recreational, household, and vocational activities, as well as self-care.

The use of METs offers the longer-living, retired aging-MBB great insight into the value of remaining physically active and demonstrates that all types of daily tasks provide a physiological training effect. Most importantly, it clearly shows those self-care activities that allow him to live independently are between 2 and 3 METs. The ability to measure this level of energy expenditure means his new goal is to find and maintain daily activities that elicit a 3 to 4 MET level of energy expenditure—as those will keep the bar from falling down to the point where he is unable to live independently.

One final point about the use of METs. The key difference between performing 3 to 4 MET level activities at age twenty-five and age sixty-five is that your maximal level of fitness has changed. When you were twenty-five, your maximal MET level was a 15, which meant those same 3 to 4 MET activities required only a minimal effort (20 to 25% of your maximal abilities). Today your maximal MET level has dropped to an 8, which means those same 3 to 4 MET activities require a much higher level of effort (40 to 50% of your max).

For those who are struggling with the math, let me provide an example. Raking leaves will always be a 5 MET activity. The reason that task seems harder at age sixty-five than at age twenty-five is because it used to require a modest 33 percent level of effort but now requires a 63 percent level of effort. Raking leaves is not impossible at age sixty-five; it is just harder to perform because your max METs have declined with aging.

The bottom line: Just because those daily tasks of our youth were not marketed as legitimate exercise does not mean they

EXAMPLES OF MET LEVELS AND EVERYDAY ACTIVITIES

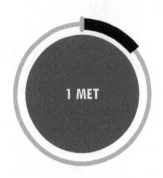

1 MET

Subject is awake and resting comfortably in a chair

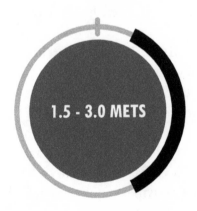

1.5 - 3.0 METS

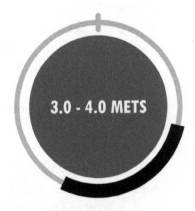

3.0 - 4.0 METS

Self-care	shaving, dressing, trimming nails
Household	setting table, light sweeping, ironing
Recreational	playing piano, billiards, bowling
Occupation	desk work, light assembly, typing

Self-care	showering, driving, climbing stairs
Household	washing floor, grocery shopping, bed making
Recreational	bodyweight calisthenics, golfing with pull cart
Occupation	light repair, painting without ladders

Running errands, performing regular household chores,
and engaging in other lifestyle tasks can be effective ways
to boost your Metabolic Equivalents (METS). While there
are differences in the metabolic cost of structured exercise
versus routine daily activities, you can see by these illustra-
tions that engaging in consistent daily activities or chores
can improve your overall health.

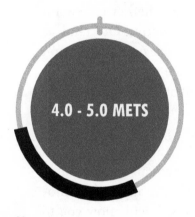

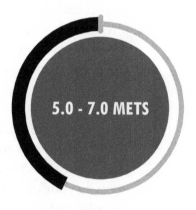

	4.0 - 5.0 METS		5.0 - 7.0 METS
Self-care	none	**Self-care**	none
Household	washing windows, pushing lawn mower, hand raking leaves	**Household**	splitting wood, putting on storm windows
Recreational	badminton, slow dancing, doubles tennis	**Recreational**	singles tennis, square dancing, stream fishing
Occupation	light farming, painting, light shoveling	**Occupation**	heavy farming, construction, climbing ladders

were not beneficial. Every form of physical activity that is above 4-5 MET's will keep you out of the Assisted Living facilities.

I offer the following suggestions to my fellow longer-living, aging-MBB who is entering the early stages of a lengthy retirement period.

- Accept the fact that we are all inactive relative to our younger days. And while we are not the first generation to go through the decline associated with the aging process, we are the first to go through a longer aging process. Every day we make decisions about the level of activity that we will be able to perform over the next ten to twenty years of our life.

- Appreciate that we get to decide whether to remain physically, mentally, and socially active. Our choices determine whether we check the *able* or *unable* box on the assisted living preadmittance questionnaire—or whether we will even have to fill out that form.

- Realize that the creative marketing labels of fit or unfit are only relevant to world-class athletes. You need to differentiate between the terms able and unable because your only goal is to remain physically, emotionally, and mentally active, which will allow you to live independently.

- Understand the significant financial savings of being able to live independently, because the cost of assisted living will be greater than any of your previous home mortgage payments.

- Pursue only those activities that allow you to maintain a positive mood, as nobody wants to visit or take care of a grumpy old man.

NOT TOO LATE

In summary, every aging-MBB has been thinking about his retirement since the day he started earning a living. Most of us view it as the next stage of our life with the hope of being able to enjoy ourselves. We also realize there is going to be a legitimate financial cost to retirement. Your financial cost will be driven by longer life expectancy and an ever-growing list of tasks that you may be unable to perform.

Your personal savings are not enough to pay for your retirement unless you choose to remain physically, emotionally, and socially engaged. The financial bottom line for every aging-MBB is to rethink how we want to spend our money and our final days. Twenty years from now, it will be easy to tell those of us who were unable to successfully plan ahead by the slogan on their T-shirt: "If I had known I was going to live this long, I would have taken much better care of myself."

It's not too late to start making a commitment to remain physically active – while you are still ABLE.

5

YOUR CHOICES, WHILE YOU'RE STILL ABLE TO MAKE HEALTHY ONES

I have always found it odd that the first step behind many of the world's legendary scientific discoveries can be traced back to a fortuitous observation, such as Sir Isaac Newton's inadvertent yet historic observations and later proof of gravity.

I have to admit I always found it ironic, but one such casual and unintended observation opened the door to the science of exercise physiology. After World War II, British health researchers noticed an unexpected increase in the rate of people dying of heart attacks. Out of curiosity, British epidemiologist Jeremy Morris set up a study to look at the rates of heart attack of people in various occupations, including school teachers, postmen, and double-decker bus drivers.

Morris had his aha moment in 1949 when he reviewed the double-decker bus data and made the connection between levels of physical activity and cardiac health. The data showed that the drivers had higher rates of heart attacks than the ticket takers. His initial observations were that the bus drivers were completely sedentary and much larger in body size while the ticket takers were not only smaller in stature but constantly climbing up and down the stairs of the bus. This observation quickly spread, and the United States began to conduct similar research regarding the relationship between levels of physical activity and coronary artery disease. Keep in mind, in 1949 heart disease was the number-one cause of death in the US—and it still is.

The idea that heart attacks could be prevented was a significant change in medicine because most medical textbooks took a single-layered approach to the definition of health. A patient was considered to be medically healthy based solely on the absence of disease. In other words, a patient was either healthy or unhealthy.

The problem for most physicians was they become increasingly aware that there were differences in the rates that genetically similar people developed heart disease, high blood pressure, obesity, and type 2 diabetes. They also noticed there were differences across different regions of the United States. These observations meant that the medical definition of health had to be broadened to consider a person's lifestyle choices and possibly their location.

This new approach meant medicine could still use a black-and-white approach to a definitive diagnosis like pregnancy (you either are or aren't), but it needed a broader spectrum of colors when diagnosing an individual's overall health status. The more comprehensive approach to diagnosing health status also proved beneficial because it was clear that Americans were living and dying in shades of gray.

One of the first US physicians who believed there had to be some measurable relationship between a person's daily lifestyle choices and health status was Lester Breslow, a physician and public health advocate. In the mid-1960s Dr. Breslow observed a difference in the everyday habits between patients previously classified as healthy and those classified as unhealthy. Specifically, he observed that healthy patients had similarities when it came to their sleep, body weight, alcohol consumption, cigarette smoking, food consumption, and levels of physical activity.

It is worth mentioning that Dr. Breslow was ahead of his time, because the structured exercise movement had not yet started;

national obesity rates had not yet begun to increase; cigarette warnings had not become mandatory; and automated technology was not viewed as having any downside.

The next step for Dr. Breslow was to statistically prove there was a legitimate cause and effect between a person's health status and their lifestyle choices. In an effort to demonstrate this connection, he took a longitudinal approach to collecting his data, which means he observed people over time.

This type of statistical approach allowed him to compare and contrast the cumulative effect of any daily habit or lifestyle choice on roughly 7,000 Americans for over twenty years. The power of longitudinal data is that the technique quantifies the long-term effect that a specific health habit has on a person's health status. Quite simply, if you want to measure the twenty-year effect that smoking a pack of cigarettes each day has on an individual's health, you need to follow that person for twenty years.

...it is never too late to change an unhealthy habit, because the human body is capable of recovering from self-imposed trauma.

The great news for today's aging male baby boomer (aging-MBB) is twofold. First, men who are able to maintain a higher number of simple-to-follow daily healthy habits will have a better quality of life. Second, it is never too late to change an unhealthy habit, because the human body is capable of recovering from self-imposed trauma. Like I said, this is great news for most men as most never really worried about the long-term health consequences of their choices when they were young. I refer to our reckless days during high school, college, and early adulthood, and no one needs to be reminded what those were like, just that we'd like to have them back for any number of reasons.

The medical community was not the only research group that believed changing human behavior could improve health status. In the late 1970s James Prochaska, a psychologist, and his colleagues began to observe five distinct steps that were needed to create successful behavior change. Their premise was that people need to move from one stage to the next when trying to change a behavior. In other words, successful long-term behavior change was more complicated than simply being told you should quit smoking. They believed that successful long-term behavior change involved a person's ability to complete all five of their stages of change, from just thinking about changing a behavior to actually doing it and maintaining the behavior over time.

The key takeaway for every aging-MBB is this: long-term behavior change is a step-by-step process. Unfortunately, man's ability to change each specific habit is not created equally. For example, a man could easily become frustrated when he notices he has a greater degree of difficulty changing a specific health habit than did his best friend, brother, or identical twin.

In the end, every aging-MBB needs to be ready, willing, and able to make a choice when it comes to improving his health status. As I mentioned in the previous chapters, the goal for every one of us is to live independently for as long as possible. The only way to attain this goal is to understand the cause and effect between everyday lifestyle choices and overall health status. Most importantly, we need to realize that we are still able to make healthy choices.

I have spent my career improving the health and fitness of a wide cross-section of Americans. These experiences have allowed me to compile a list of twelve lifestyle choices that all began as observations (maybe not as profound as Newton's) and later were shown to have a beneficial cause and effect specific to the male baby boomer. Keep in mind my twelve habits will not change your mortality, but as Lee Marvin convinced his twelve dirty dozen soldiers, you still have the opportunity to change the course of the rest of your life.

you still have the opportunity to change the course of the rest of your life.

Given that introduction, the following is what I refer to as a healthier and cleaner dirty dozen. It is my hope that you will choose to adopt them into your everyday lifestyle.

DAN'S HEALTHY DIRTY DOZEN

(1) THROW AWAY THE CIGARETTES

Remember how popular cigarette smoking was in the 1950s and 1960s American culture? The Marlboro man was displayed on roadside billboards across the country. Dean Martin and Johnny Carson openly smoked cigarettes on their weekly prime time television shows. Frank Sinatra made singing with a cigarette in one hand and a microphone in the other hand an art form. Make no mistake about it, at its peak in popularity, smoking a cigarette was as cool as it got!

To this day, I am still amazed at the number of people who fail to accept the direct cause-and-effect relationship between smoking cigarettes and lung cancer. It seems every aging-MBB who still smokes cigarettes justifies why he started and why he continues to smoke.

I have tested numerous military veterans who explained that the only reason they smoke is because they started in boot camp when the government included cigarettes in their K-rations. I've heard other smokers say, "I started when I went to bars and restaurants with friends in my late teens," or "I started as a sort of rebellion against people who viewed me as a quiet kid with no sense of direction." Each of these groups had one thing in common—they clearly remembered when or why they started. They just never got around to quitting.

My earliest introduction to athletes or fitness-conscious people who smoked cigarettes was with the National Hockey League (NHL). Prior to graduate school, I worked for a very successful group of athletic clubs in Minneapolis. At that time, the Minnesota North Stars were the town's NHL team and some team members would visit the club. Turns out, smoking cigarettes was not frowned upon in the NHL, because it didn't limit the hockey player's ability to skate and gave the players something to do between game periods and after the game.

Countless other fitness members who smoked would smugly remind me that their smoking habit was the reason they started running (as if running somehow would cancel the harmful effects of the smoking). What makes this even more confusing is that most of these people were actually quite fit. Sadly, most of those runners will continue to run until they get a terminal diagnosis of emphysema or throat or lung cancer—which is something they can't outrun.

I had a big wake-up call when my wife and I were on vacation in Maui. We had just walked off the hotel property down a pathway toward the ocean when the couple in front of us abruptly stopped to apply some sunscreen. As we walked around them, I overheard the conversation: "Make sure you use the one with the strongest SPF rating." As for my wake-up call, I noticed that the person demanding the highest SPF factor to prevent skin cancer was smoking a cigarette.

Every aging-MBB needs to accept the CDC's cause-and-effect research regarding the health risks associated with smoking cigarettes. The research-based facts are undeniable:

- More than ten times as many US citizens have died prematurely from smoking cigarettes than have died in all the wars fought by the United States during its history.

- 480,000 people in the United States die every year from illness caused by smoking cigarettes.

- Smoking causes about 90 percent of all lung cancer deaths.

- Smoking causes about 80 percent of all deaths from chronic obstructive pulmonary disease (COPD).

- Quitting smoking for two to five years cuts your risk of stroke to about the same as nonsmokers.

- Quitting smoking for ten years cuts your risk of developing lung cancer in half.

A lot of people have given me credit for helping them achieve some level of fitness. Ironically, I am convinced the greatest and most sincere compliment I get is from people who say I helped them stop smoking. I say that because it's easy for nonsmokers to forget that the nicotine in cigarettes is a highly addictive drug—a drug that doesn't require a prescription to purchase, nor is it illegal to use. Nicotine needs to be viewed in a similar fashion to other addictive drugs in that most people fail to quit using it without some type of outside intervention program.

As a nonsmoking aging-MBB, I no longer attempt to discuss the dangers of smoking cigarettes with smokers for two reasons. The first is nobody has ever said, "Thanks for telling me about the health risks associated with smoking. I never knew it was bad for me," and, second, smoking cigarettes is an addiction and should be addressed by professionals who deal with drug addictions.

I now offer just one bit of advice to my fellow male boomers who currently smoke or who ask me how to help someone who is struggling to quit smoking. I tell them to watch the PBS American Masters series on Johnny Carson. The show is about two hours long and highlights the career of a true television legend. The last ten minutes of the show are especially poignant, because his friends and family discuss how even Carson had to finally accept that his emphysema was due to his smoking. The most powerful segment was from one of his closest friends when recalling his last conversation with Johnny saying, "It was those damn cigarettes."

The best news for every aging-MBB regarding cigarette smoking is it's never too late to quit and never too late to ask for help. If you are still struggling to quit, you should consider the destructive health consequences you are causing others via your secondhand smoke.

I have included a list of successful stop smoking programs on the www.danielzeman.com website.

② GET REGULAR PREVENTIVE MEDICAL EXAMS

I grew up in Rochester, Minnesota, home of the world-famous Mayo Clinic. My mother was a nurse who worked at Mayo, which meant I was constantly being introduced to physicians up until the day I left for college.

Fast-forward a few years and it was a physician who offered me my first real job inside St. Mary's Hospital in Minneapolis. As expected, I worked with physicians there. Later on, my days at the Minneapolis Sports Medicine Center meant I was introduced to yet another group of physicians. It is safe to say, I knew the names and phone numbers of plenty of physicians.

But from age twenty-five to forty-five, the only phone number I dialed when I had a real emergency belonged to Jim Nelson. Jim Nelson was not a physician. He was and remains the best auto mechanic that I ever met, and he never failed me in a real-life crisis. I called Jim Nelson because he could make a diagnosis over the phone and he was never wrong.

Each of our phone calls started with me in a panic saying, "I woke up this morning and my car just didn't sound right," or "I was driving along, and all of a sudden my car just felt sluggish," or "My car just started leaking something all over the garage floor." He would assure me by saying,

"Sounds like a fuel problem," or "Got to be something with your pressure," or "Your seals are getting old and everything begins to leak."

All I knew was if I drove my car into his shop, he would put it up on the lift or look under the hood, and in a matter of minutes the mystery problem would be cured. He would also make sure to check the other vital signs, and, if need be, he scheduled my car for its next routine maintenance checkup.

However, the greatest lesson I learned from Jim Nelson was the day I noticed a car in his shop that appeared to be in great physical shape, but when I asked what was wrong with it, he said, "It's bad news, the owner never had routine checkups, he just kept driving it after the red warning light was flashing, so now he has to decide if he can afford to fix it or if he should just junk it."

Jim Nelson convinced me that performing routine preventive maintenance saved me money. Things like rotating the tires or changing the motor oil were relatively inexpensive, and they allowed me to avoid paying future costly repairs bills. I also expanded my commitment to perform routine preventive maintenance on my home including the furnace, air conditioner, refrigerator, and computers. To this day, I always methodically stick to a routine maintenance schedule on all of my possessions because I am convinced it increases their efficiency and saves me money.

My reason for mentioning Jim Nelson should be obvious to you now. One of the great ironies in preventive medicine is that men will perform routine maintenance on cars and air conditioners, but they will not schedule preventive medical checkups on their bodies that they know can't be replaced.

What makes matters worse, the analogies are so obvious that it only adds to the ignorance of men's behavior. Consider these examples.

- A man knows the ideal viscosity for the engine oil in his car that will keep the engine from burning up, yet he does not monitor the viscosity of the fats in his blood that keeps his human heart from overheating.

- He gladly pays to have a technician remove the clogs in his home's furnace ventilation tubing, yet he doesn't have the same enthusiasm about having his colon checked for similar blockages.

- He knows the ideal tire pressure for his automobiles to avoid blowouts that could lead to deadly crashes, yet he does not monitor his blood pressure that can increase his risk of deadly or traumatic strokes.

- He performs yearly battery replacements on home carbon monoxide systems that allow him to track the levels of this invisible killer, yet he does not monitor his PSA levels that allow him to track for prostate cancer—a condition that is more than a whispering concern for every man.

- Finally, he is constantly on a search-and-destroy mission for a growing list of new computer viruses, yet he does not approach the oldest human viruses like influenza or pneumonia with the same level of aggression.

I believe our generational timeline offers some insight into why men lack a desire to maintain regular visits to physicians. Our lack of medical screening started in our youth based on the medical fact that, as a group, nothing can really go wrong.

For those of us who did have early medical screenings, our strongest memories involved the dreaded instructional phrase to "turn your head and cough." The key difference is these mandatory exams cleared us to play high school sports and were part of military entrance exams or job acceptance, but they were not designed to prevent or minimize the risk of getting injured, becoming sick, or dying prematurely.

Every aging-MBB has heard about the need to begin a regular medical screening program yet most continue to avoid making an appointment. I have found the biggest reason why men eventually make an appointment to get screened is after a close friend was diagnosed with a terminal illness. In essence, men still find fear rather than logic to be the greatest incentive to begin a regular program of preventive medical screens.

The CDC says these easy-to-schedule annual appointments will reduce your risk of developing deadly diseases by tracking your key biological markers, keeping you vaccinated against preventable diseases such as shingles and pneumonia, and outlining a sensible plan based on your family history. Checkups and screenings can help catch a host of diseases early—when they are more easily treatable. Consider this list of diseases and their simple screenings.

- Cancer—early detection saves lives
  - ▶ Lung via LDCT screening for current or previous smokers
  - ▶ Colon via colonoscopy or flexible sigmoidoscopy
  - ▶ Skin via mole observation or biopsy
  - ▶ Prostate via blood draw (PSA level) and physical exam

- Heart Disease—early management saves lives
  - ▶ Via blood draw to measure cholesterol, HDL, LDL, triglyceride levels
  - ▶ Via treadmill test (walking or running with EKG monitor)

- Diabetes—minimizing spikes in blood glucose saves lives
  - ▶ Via blood draw to measure glucose, hemoglobin A1C levels

- Stroke—lowering blood pressure saves lives
  - ▶ Via blood pressure screening

- Family History—identifying genetic tendencies improves lives
  - ▶ Via one-on-one discussion with a healthcare professional about family health history

- Virus—vaccinations save lives and reduce complications
  - ▶ Via immunization shots for influenza (annual), shingles, pneumonia

- Depression—accepting the diagnosis improves quality of lives
  - ▶ Via simple Q&A with healthcare professional

Initially all of the preventive medical test scores can be overwhelming, but it's important to know your medical test scores and numbers and what they mean. As I see it, if you are able to instantly recall your four-digit pin and your nine-digit social security number, then you can remember your blood pressure and cholesterol.

The first step for every aging-MBB is to take the time to find a physician (primary care or internist) with whom you can openly discuss each of the possible medical screening procedures. Keep in mind, every physician has already heard every question, concern, or fear that you feel is holding you back. You and your physician should agree on an annual screening schedule and do not forget to include screenings for vision, hearing, and dental, as these three are often neglected but still have a significant effect on your overall health status.

Today, I still call my life-saving mechanic Jim Nelson whenever I have an emergency with my car. However, I also have the phone number of my primary care physician on speed dial. The bottom line for every aging-MBB is to avoid being the guy whom Jim Nelson would say, "That guy's car is being hauled off to permanent recycling, because he kept driving it even when the warning light was flashing." In other words, I call my physician because this doc helps me maintain my overall health status, which should be every aging-MBB's most cherished possession.

Finally, I would like every aging-MBB to rethink the differences between his health insurance and his automobile insurance. Keep in mind both of these insurance providers are designed to pay out less money than they accumulate in premiums. Stated more bluntly, both are for-profit businesses.

Originally, automobile insurance allowed you to be financially prepared for the scenario of your car needing emergency repairs caused by an accident or unavoidable occurrence. The two fundamental truths that allow automobile insurance providers to remain profitable are, one, automobile insurance does not pay for preventive maintenance, and, second, every automobile has a decreasing value. In other words, Jim Nelson does not accept my auto insurance card as payment for my oil changes, and I will never get an insurance check that is greater than the value of my aging car.

By the same token, health insurance originally allowed you to be financially prepared for the occasional broken bone, surprise appendectomy, or any other emergency medical occurrence. However, the landscape changed after medicine created numerous life-saving and life-extending treatments. The new dilemma for every aging-MBB is believing his insurance provider should be responsible to pay for every new medical treatment across his generation's longer life-span. The reality is that health insurance does not pay for everything. Keep in mind, the healthcare insurance providers are designed to be profitable. As of yet, this relatively new scenario shows no sign of being solved.

I have used the analogy to compare health insurance and automobile insurance for many years when doing talks about the importance of preventive medical screening. Primarily because the majority of men understand they have a responsibility to maintain their automobiles. I have also found that before I drive away, a member of the audience stops and shares a common story about one of their children. Each begins by saying their son or daughter called and needs money to pay for some problem with their car. They usually say their child's automobile "needs a new battery" or "needs a new motor" or "needs a new radiator."

I have learned to quickly interject and ask, "Did you give them the money?" to which they reply, "Yes, but they have to pay me back because I am not paying for their neglect."

I then ask, "Can you imagine what would happen to our automobile insurance rates if our providers were forced to cover the cost of every driver's—the young and the old—decision to neglect and abuse their automobiles?" As expected the immediate responses include "the rates would skyrocket" or "they can't afford to fix every car" or "that's why they blue book values on cars."

I have three suggestions to every longer-living, aging-MBB.

1. Accept we are all going to be that car with high mileage due to our advanced ages and some of us have neglected to perform routine medical maintenance.

2. Understand that elderly humans do not have a decreasing blue book value.

3. Remember, affordable health insurance is based on
    the ability to minimize medical claims or to spread
    the cost of healthcare across a larger group of future
    (healthier) payers.

If we struggle with these three concepts, then we will force
someone—the government or the insurance providers—to
make decisions as to how much health insurance money can
be allocated to the aging-MBB and which medical problems
are justifiably worth fixing.

I believe the legacy of the male baby boomer will not
be that we lived longer than other generations of men. It
will be whether or not we expected future generations to
pay for our decision to avoid scheduling preventive medical
screens. In reality, somebody will eventually have to pay for
our medical expenses. We have the personal and financial
responsibility to take care of our health. The ability to minimize our long-term medical care begins with taking personal
responsibility for maintaining a regular schedule of preventive
medical screenings.

My suggestion to every aging-MBB who is struggling
to schedule medical screening is to understand that you,
not your insurance provider, has the most to gain or lose
if you stay healthier. I encourage you to identify the single
greatest piece of equipment in your garage, tool shed, or
home and compare its longevity and relative importance to
your own body.

Each of us will eventually realize that our body is the
most complicated, self-regulating, and interactive piece of
equipment you own. It was with you when you took your
first breath of air, your first step, and your body has allowed
you to get up after your first fall. It allowed you to solve your
first math problem, speak your first sentence, and sing your
first song. It allowed you to stand up for what you believed

in and bend over to help those who needed help. In return it deserves a regular schedule of tune-ups and checkups, which will allow you to enjoy every chance you get to be in the driver's seat of your life's journey.

I have included a list of the recommended preventive medical screens for the aging MBB on the www.danielzeman.com website.

(3) DETERMINE A HEALTHY-LIVING WEIGHT

How much should you weigh? That's a long-standing medical debate. The answer is "it depends!"

Certainly, a person's age, gender, nationality, height, stage of physical development, and professional occupation play a part in identifying a person's ideal weight. The key for every aging-MBB is to recalculate his ideal body weight with the goal of living independently as long as possible. His ability to maintain a healthy body weight throughout the aging process means greater mobility, agility, and stamina, as well as reducing the need for walking aids, prescription medications, or the future need for assisted care.

Your body weight can easily be measured using any bathroom scale, but the ability to measure your body composition provides greater insight into your overall health status. The aging process has been shown to decrease muscle mass and bone density, as well as lead to an increase in fat storage, so it's important to measure these ever-changing variables when calculating an ideal healthy-living weight.

The early science behind determining a healthy weight for a male was based on three variables: his height, frame size, and visual amount of muscularity. The basic belief was that men with larger frame sizes who appeared more muscular would be allowed to weigh more than those who had a smaller frame size with less muscularity.

It is important to remember this timeline demanded men to be very physically active, and they were not expected to live very long. In other words, there wasn't a need for medicine to pursue a cause-and-effect relationship between a man's body weight and his long-term health or if having excess body weight causes an increased risk of damage to his ankles, hips, or knees. Men simply died before those factors would have made a difference in his longevity or health during his later years.

Fortunately, medical advancements, updated technology, and increases in life expectancy have forced a change in the approach to determining how much a man should weigh. The real challenge was to show why two men with similar sized frames could weigh the same but have significantly different risks of developing life-threatening diseases. The new variable was found to be his amount of fat tissue, so we need to determine if a man was overweight or overfat.

In the late 1940s, Albert Behnke, a physician, began developing body composition testing procedures. His test involved weighing people underwater and incorporating the science of Archimedes's principle of buoyancy. Later, W. E. Siri and J. Brozek expanded Dr. Behnke's research and collectively introduced a type of whole-body density testing known as hydrostatic or underwater weighing. Since the density of human body fat was known, it was now possible to use a person's whole-body density to calculate their percentage of body fat.

I have underwater weighed countless people, and I start each test explaining the science behind testing for body density and body volume. I begin saying, "The easiest way to explain the science of measuring body density via underwater weighing is for you to imagine weighing a five-pound rock and a five-pound life preserver under water. Remember both weigh the same on the bathroom scale, but when I put the rock in the water, it will instantly sink to the bottom of the tank. When I put the life jacket in the tank, it will float on top of the water. Today we are going to find out if your body will float like the life jacket due to a higher percentage of fat or if it will sink like the rock due to a higher percentage of denser tissue—like muscle and bones."

Next, I discuss the science of testing for body volume. Once again, the rock and life jacket scenario make this an easy visual. I continue by saying, "The other thing to notice about the five-pound rock and life jacket is their difference in size. The rock is about the size of a small brick, but the life jacket is much larger and fluffier than the rock because of its lack of density. These measurable differences in body volume are why most people can weigh the same as they did in high school but can no longer wear the same size pants—as those no longer fit, especially around the waist!"

I have also measured the body composition on numerous professional athletes, including players from the Minnesota Vikings and Minnesota Timberwolves. The main difference is professional athletes do not use percent body fat testing to determine how much fat they have. Instead, each athlete uses it to determine their ideal playing weight. The idea that athletes have ideal playing weight is based on the connection between athletic performance measures such as vertical jump, quickness, agility, strength, cardiovascular endurance, and the player's body weight—or their scale weight.

Underwater weighing calculates each athlete's body weight as the sum of two components: their fat pounds and their LBM (lean body mass). Originally the thought was to make sure each athlete had the lowest number of fat pounds and the highest amount of lean body mass. The last twenty-five years have shown me that this single-focused approach does not always provide each athlete with his ideal playing weight. For example, a player can become so focused on having and keeping the least amount of fat that he is constantly underfed. This means he can no longer maintain intense training routines because he does not have enough calories on board to use as fuel.

I have also found athletes who become so focused on maintaining the most amount of lean body mass that they are constantly spending hours lifting weights. This means they do not have enough time during the week to spend on improving their sport-specific performance skills.

The single goal of every professional athlete is peak performance. An athlete's ideal playing weight equals the sum of the optimal number of fat pounds and the optimal number for lean body mass that matches his peak performance. My recommendation to the aging-MBB is to use the same two-component approach when you try to identify an ideal healthy-living weight.

The CDC is a reputable source that shows the increased risks for various diseases for an overweight or obese person. Men who are overweight are at increased risk of developing or being diagnosed with these diseases:

- Type 2 diabetes

- High blood pressure (hypertension)

- Coronary artery disease due to increased levels of LDL cholesterol and triglycerides

- Stroke

- Sleep apnea

- Cancer of colon, liver, kidney, gallbladder

- Mental illness such as depression or anxiety

The good news for the aging-MBB is the CDC has also shown each of these increased health risks can be reduced when you lose body weight.

The biggest drawback in these studies is the majority of them did not measure or use fat pounds but only used body weight. This flaw does not diminish the research or make their findings less valid, but it makes it difficult to show individualized outcomes. Today, it is well known that all weight loss or gain is not the same. For example, two men can both lose twenty pounds on the bathroom scale, but one loses significantly more of the weight from his fat pounds while the other loses much more of his weight from his lean body mass.

I have tested many men who mistakenly believed they needed to lose twenty-five to thirty pounds to achieve a healthy weight. After measuring their body fat levels and beginning a sensible weight loss program, they found losing as few as ten to fifteen pounds of body fat was all that was needed to have a significant reduction in their systolic blood pressure, cholesterol, triglycerides, or blood glucose levels. The key is they lost those pounds of fat.

Men who are able to understand the relationship between their fat weight and their health seem to have a much easier time maintaining an ideal healthy-living weight. For example, some will say, "I have found that if I can keep my weight under 185 pounds, my blood pressure stays low and I just feel better." They further explain, "I could lose another five to seven pounds of fat and get down to 178 to 180, but it doesn't continue to lower my blood pressure or alter how I feel—plus, it means that I have to be so much more focused on counting calories and my eating habits, which makes my life so rigid."

In essence, these men are like the professional athlete who realizes he could continue to strive to lose more body fat but doing so doesn't improve his peak performance. Every aging-MBB needs to realize that his ability to perform—stay healthy—is now based on his ability to monitor health measures such as blood pressure, blood sugar, and blood lipid levels (cholesterol is one). The ability to measure each of these variables and contrast them against his number of fat pounds allows him to arrive at the optimal number of fat pounds that are part of his healthy-living weight.

This scenario is why sports medicine groups have suggested using 18 to 22 percent body fat as the ideal body fat range where the aging-MBB will receive the greatest health benefits. They are not saying it is not possible to achieve an even lower percentage of body fat; rather, they do not find it to be any more beneficial.

The final calculation for determining an ideal healthy-living weight is to understand the importance of maintaining the correct amount of lean body mass. Every aging-MBB needs to understand his ability to maintain or minimize the loss of lean body mass (LBM) as he ages is one of the keys to living independently.

The medical profession classifies the loss of LBM in terms of two critical subcategories: muscle mass and bone density.

The projected loss of muscle mass for every aging-MBB is 10 percent per decade starting at age fifty. The loss of LBM is generally considered to be naturally occurring and driven by the brain's inability to communicate with the skeletal muscles, as well as lower concentrations of growth hormone and testosterone. However, researchers have shown that elderly men who maintain a regular resistance training program can alter the loss of muscle mass.

The ability to consistently project the expected loss of bone density in aging men is more difficult because a man's behavior plays a greater role than nature. For example, smoking and too much alcohol combined with not enough sunshine and inadequate vitamin D or calcium consumption can accelerate the loss of bone density. Once again, strength training is beneficial to maintaining bone density, but its impact is limited by the factors I just listed.

The bottom line for every aging-MBB is to consistently measure the loss of LBM (muscle mass or bone density) as it impacts peak strength and muscle endurance and reduces the risks of falls and bone fractures.

If you want to stay on the playing field of life for as long as possible, identify and maintain a healthy ideal playing weight. Monitoring the number of fat pounds will provide insight into the risk of developing diseases, while monitoring lean body mass will provide insight into your ability to maintain your strength, mobility, and agility that will allow you to live independently.

The good news is that body composition testing continues to be more common within the medical community and can be included in your yearly medical screening routine. Just talk with your physician about the testing.

The following case study represents an ideal scenario (taken from medical notes) for the aging-MBB.

Subject: a 5 foot 9 inch, 65-year-old male, weighing 200 lbs. was seen due to complaints of increasing levels of daily fatigue and borderline hypertension. He was found to have 25% fat using an underwater weighing test. These results determined that he has 50 lbs. of body fat and 150 lbs. of LBM. The subject chose to use the 18-22% body fat recommendations as a means of determining a healthy-living weight. Using this method his new body weight range was calculated to be between 183-192 lbs. or he needed to lose 8-17 lbs. of fat. The patient agreed to begin an exercise program and dietary changes that would lead to a loss of 8 pounds of fat and would return in 6 months to contrast his blood pressure, level of fatigue and total fat pounds. As a point of reference, the Metropolitan height/weight charts would recommend a new ideal weight for him to be 148-160 lbs. or 155-176 lbs. depending on his frame size being considered medium or large.

As I mentioned, that case study represents the ideal scenario for the aging-MBB. The patient was given objective data about his body weight and encouraged to return and see the effect that losing eight pounds of body fat could have on his health status. In essence, it removes the emotional attachment or preconceived beliefs that a man's body weight is not that big a health risk. Certainly, we all know men who are fatter than we are and they all seem to be very happy.

I wrote this book as an educational wake-up call for every aging-MBB. In other words, I did not write it to educate you on how to be happy today, but rather to educate you on how your current habits will impact your level of health and happiness throughout your longer-than-expected life. The following professional and personal insights should provide the motivation to rethink the negative effect of having excess body weight across the aging process.

Today's retired professional male athlete provides the best example of the cumulative effect that body weight has on his long-term mobility. The majority of professional athletes' careers are cut short by knee or other joint injuries prior to age thirty. Sadly, most of these career-ending skeletal injuries will continue to cause them varying degrees of limitations for the rest of their lives. The longer-living, aging-MBB needs to understand his skeletal system is capable of suffering the same damage. The destructive effect on the knee joint of the NBA basketball player will occur quicker (earlier in life), but the same knee damage will be seen on the aging-MBB due to the cumulative effect that excess weight has on his knees. It really is just a matter of direct force over a period of time.

The exponential rise in the number of total knee replacements should provide us with insight into the similar conversation these guys will have with an orthopedic surgeon. The thirty-year-old professional athlete and the seventy-year-old retired, overweight grandfather will both hear, "Sorry your knee just wasn't meant to support that type of abuse."

The only difference is the overweight seventy-year-old will be informed prior to his optional knee replacement surgery that losing weight before his surgery will improve his surgical outcome. Biomechanics data shows a 6:1 ratio of actual body weight to true resistance. For example, if you were to lose 20 pounds on the scale, you would really be losing 120 pounds (6x20) of real exertion on the knee joint for every step you take. Not surprising, the majority of NBA teams have begun to control playing minutes of their athletes as they realize it reduces impact on knees, hips, and ankles.

Another relevant example of the problems with excessive fat weight comes from thoracic surgeons. In these cases, the main difference is where the excess body fat is stored or accumulates. In our youth, the majority of excess fat calories were stored subcutaneously or directly under the skin. This is why the original "pinch an inch" advertisement made sense because you literally could pinch the excess fat. However, the aging process has directed more of the excess fat to be stored inside the body as what is called intra-abdominal fat. This new storage location is of concern to the thoracic surgeons because it interferes with their ability to successfully perform surgeries around the heart, liver, and gallbladder.

Keep in mind, this is now a legitimate concern to every longer-living, aging-MBB because the longer he lives, the more likely he will need one or more of these surgical procedures.

Finally regarding ideal weight, I have one personal insight as to why we need to understand the impact and the consequences of dealing with excess weight. Let me warn you, it has nothing to do with body fat, but for the last twenty-five years I have used it in every talk I have given on the consequences of excess body fat, and every audience has found it insightful.

I decided to attend graduate school when I realized that I needed a formal education if I was going to improve the health of the unhealthy. I also realized it meant selling the majority of my belongings and packing everything else into a U-Haul trailer, as well as installing a trailer hitch to my 1978 Cutlass. I left Minneapolis with some cash, a map, and budget that should have allowed me enough of a buffer to arrive within two to three days of travel to Texas.

I had a huge wake-up call before I hit the Iowa state line. My Cutlass was literally eating gasoline. I thought there had to be a hole in the gas tank. I instantly had to rethink my travel plans as to how far I could go between gas stations. I didn't know how many miles I could go before my engine would just run out of fuel. The good news is I eventually arrived in Texas, but I learned a simple yet valuable lesson about the consequences of pulling extra weight around. If you are trying to minimize the wear and tear on the engine and tires and get the best gas mileage, then unhook the U-Haul you're pulling.

Total body weight dictates the workload placed on every one of our internal organs, skeletal muscles, and tendons inside our body. Similar to the professional athlete, you have the ability to determine a healthy-living weight by redefining your ideal number of fat pounds and lean body mass that will ensure a peak performance as you battle (and win) the aging process. It really gets down to simple math of your body's ability to successfully tolerate unnecessary forces (extra weight) across an extended period of time (longer life expectancy).

I have included a method of measuring your percentage of body fat on the www.danielzeman.com website.

4) SAFETY MEASURES AREN'T JUST FOR KIDS

Every aging-MBB grew up hearing some version of the motto, "Things that don't kill you will make you stronger." The idea that we should approach life with some degree of caution regarding our personal safety was definitely not part of our generation's philosophy.

As infants, we were never cautiously snapped into car seats. Instead, most of us preferred lying on top of the back-seat under the rear window and we loved it. As toddlers, we ate whatever our parents or older siblings put in front of us proclaiming, "Try it, you'll like it."

As adolescents, we either jumped or fell off any tree or fence post we climbed up. For those who played sports, the list of things we should not have done grew exponentially. The ability to consider the safety risks of any of our activities did not improve as we entered our high school years. "Nothing good ever happens after midnight" was the only safety motto preached in the homes of every aging-MBB. As for our college experiences, I'm sure every one of us would agree there were nights when we had no idea how we made it back to the dorm safely.

Another lack of concern for personal safety for the male boomer involved reading warning labels as it was also never part of our modus operandi. This tradition continues today, as most of us forgo reading the instruction manuals of any-thing we buy. We prefer to simply plug it into the electrical wall socket and push the power button or, worse, fill it full of gas and pull the power cord.

It is safe to say the idea of personal safety has never been a priority for the male baby boomer, which explains why the number-three cause of death for men between the ages of fifty-five and sixty-four is unintentional injuries. Stated more bluntly, more men in this age group die from unintentional injuries than from liver disease, respiratory disease, diabetes, stroke, suicide, septicemia, or kidney disease combined. In fact, the cause of death for men even older—between the ages of sixty-five and upward—from unintentional injury has never dropped below number seven on their list.

The truth is every aging-MBB needs to change his mind-set about thinking he is Superman and realize he is not even Clark Kent. The things we were always told would make us stronger are now killing us.

So what are these unintentional injuries that are killing us older guys? Falls (55%), motor vehicle crashes (14%), suffocation (8%), poisoning (4%), fire (2%), and unspecified (10%). Let's look at these causes in a little more depth.

While you could say our extended aging process has made all of us more susceptible to these types of unintentional deaths, it doesn't rule out the scenarios where our stupidity or ignorance gets the best of us. So, falls, for example, can occur because the aging process brings about a natural loss in physical agility, coordination, and balance. The ability to climb stairs or ladders while simultaneously carrying suitcases and cans of paint only increases the risk of falling.

The risk of motor vehicle accidents increases due to slower reaction times, a loss of hand-eye coordination, and poor night vision. These limitations become more concerning when driving on slippery streets, during rush hour, and while attempting to use handheld phones on unfamiliar roads.

Suffocation, poisoning, and fire are often caused by poor judgment. Those who die from suffocation are often found passed out drunk in a body position where their airways are completely restricted. Poisonings are often the result of prescription drug abuse, including painkillers. Deaths by fire often occur because of lapsed judgment or forgetfulness such as home smoke detectors with dead batteries or after falling asleep in bed while smoking.

The real tragedy is that most of these deaths could have been prevented, but carelessness, poor judgment, or ignorance of the aging process played a role in why these lives were cut short.

My suggestion for every aging-MBB is to take the time and learn how to minimize your risk of unintentional accidents and injuries. We don't need to hear another disheartening story about a Vietnam veteran who survived the horrors of that war only to come home and drown on a calm lake because he wasn't wearing a life jacket or about a guy with phenomenal levels of muscular strength who died in a car accident because he didn't have the strength to snap on his seat belt.

Keep in mind that all of these scenarios are just as likely to end up causing lifelong permanent disability as they are to cause the loss of life. In either case, your loved ones will have to accept the fact that your death could have been prevented, or, worse, they will be forced into assisting with your lifelong daily medical care. Either way, the consequences of your choices are painful to you and to your loved ones who are left to pick up the pieces.

We are not the first generation of men who failed to understand the consequences of neglecting our personal safety. In fact, men have always preferred to brag about close calls with death. How often have you heard a group of guys sharing stories that end with, "I was lucky I didn't get killed," or "I'm not sure how I survived," or "Just walked away with a few scratches"?

Consider this conversation I had with a fellow male boomer. Chuck had heard about my book and asked me about its content.

I explained, "I wrote it for aging male boomers like us as an educational wake-up call about how to live independently for as long as possible." I went on to explain some of the chapters and about my recommendation for introducing twelve daily habits.

Chuck listened and then shared how he had just returned from his yearly medical exam. He said, "When I was getting ready to leave the doctor's office, he asked me about my plans for the weekend. I told him I was debating about climbing up on the roof of my house and cleaning out the gutters."

He went on, "My doc said he had been in practice for many, many years and had a very large patient population. But he said he had three male patients who are forced to live the remainder of their lives in wheelchairs. He said they all had one thing in common: they all decided they should clean their gutters."

I included that conversation because it allows each of us to see ourselves in the mirror. Did any of these guys, Chuck included, simply forget that climbing up on a roof and spraying a garden hose was going to be extremely slippery, or that having to climb up and down to move the ladder was a safer choice than trying to over-stretch their arms, or that buying a flimsy ladder to clean the gutters was a costly mistake?

I now find the term unintentional when used in front of the words cause of death or cause of injury to be rather simplistic as it implies the person didn't know any better or wasn't aware of the consequences. I think we are aware, and we're surely smarter about things that kill us. The goal is to continue to enjoy being active but to remove the word unintentional from the story line.

I have included examples of how to avoid injury when performing a variety of daily activities on the www.danielzeman.com website.

5) SLEEPING IS RECOVERING

Shortly after legendary cyclist Greg LeMond retired from cycling, I took him to a local Minneapolis fitness center. I wanted Greg to see the hottest trend in the fitness industry, as it involved cycling. The trend was called spinning—a group approach to exercising on stationary bikes. Greg took the class, and I waited to get his overall impressions of the instructor, use of music, design of the bikes, and the atmosphere created by the group of highly motivated but still novice cyclists.

As we drove away from the fitness center, his first words were, "Why doesn't the instructor understand the importance of recovery?" His comment was based on the instructor's inability to match the length of the rest interval after each intense sprinting interval. For example, there were many times when the instructor told the group, "For the next thirty seconds I want you to pedal as hard and fast as you can—an all-out sprint," but then after only a ten-second recovery period would once again demand another thirty-second all-out sprint.

Greg went on to explain that an all-out thirty-second sprint could not be followed by another similar effort if only given a ten-second recovery. I pointed out the only goal of the one-hour class was to cause intense fatigue.

I have designed a variety of intense interval-type exercise programs for a diverse group of elite athletes. It has been my experience that these athletes do not fear the brutal intensity or the fatigue that follows a day of intense training, as long as they are confident that the long-term goal is to improve peak performance. The simple physiological truth is without the correct recovery period between alternating bouts of intense efforts, there will be no long-term performance improvement—just complete fatigue.

The Tour de France (TDF) bike race offers additional insight into the need for recovery, because it demands the cyclists to be fit for the entire month of racing. In essence, the TDF can only be won by the cyclist who can balance the intensity of each day's racing with the amount of rest needed across the entire month.

This concept of balancing intensity versus recovery is nothing new to every aging-MBB as he tries to balance a hard day's work with the correct amount of recovery—and we call that sleep. Of course, the main difference is the TDF riders need to stay focused for one month while the aging-MBB's race lasts his entire lifetime.

The great news is medical research continues to highlight the benefits of regular and deep sleep. Let us accept the CDC's research highlights regarding our need for sleep and the health risks associated with not getting enough sleep.

- 35 percent of US adults do not get enough sleep

- Key sleep disorders are
  ► Insomnia—inability to initiate or maintain sleep
  ► Narcolepsy—excessive daytime sleepiness
  ► Restless Legs Syndrome—"creeping" sensation in the lower legs
  ► Sleep Apnea—interruption in regular breathing during sleep

- Adults who fail to get at least seven hours of restful sleep have
  ► Increased risk of obesity, diabetes, high blood pressure, coronary heart disease, stroke, and mental distress
  ► Impaired cognitive performance, which increases the likelihood of motor vehicle accidents

Remember those days of our youth when we could stay out all night and still wake up refreshed? Obviously, we are no longer young, which means we, like the aging professional athlete, need more time in our recovery phase. Our brain, skeletal muscles, and fluid states all need longer periods of time to recover before we can once again perform any task at the same level of effort or exertion.

Worse, some aging-MBBs believe being tired is nothing more than a state of mind, and, for them, quickly downing a Red Bull makes them good to go.

Once again, the professional athlete offers great insight into the need for adequate recovery via sleep. Research has shown the early signs of being over-trained are changes in mood states or sleep cycles. Athletes who become over-trained will begin to notice a drop-off in performance and say they feel they've "lost their competitive edge" or "feel slow." The most common rehab treatment for these athletes involves a significant reduction in their training and mandatory rest days. In other words, the new goal is to get them back to their regular sleep schedules.

Today, the best advice on proper sleep is to be consistent and go to bed at the same time each night. Get eight full hours of sleep, make sure your bedroom is quiet and relaxing, remove televisions, smartphones, and computers from the bedroom, and avoid consuming large meals, caffeine, and alcohol before bedtime.

The good news is that we can begin to feel better if we improve our sleep habits. Try this: think back to a morning when you woke up feeling rested and eager to start the new day. These restful and optimistic mornings were only possible because you were able to recover from the previous day's activities. In essence, you matched the correct recovery time to the previous day's level of intense exertion.

The motivation to begin getting a good night's sleep is simple. View your extended life expectancy as an opportunity to find enjoyment spending time doing the things that you always dreamed of doing. Your best chance of starting each morning off feeling refreshed and energized is to understand the value of recovery from the previous day's efforts.

I have included additional information on improving your sleep habits on the www.danielzeman.com website.

6 MAINTAIN MALE FRIENDSHIPS

Harry Truman is often credited with the quote, "If you want a friend in Washington, get a dog." The intent has relevance to every one of us. If you want someone who will wait at the front door when you come home, never tell you that you're wrong, never challenge your thoughts about your future, and always believe that you're perfect, then get a dog.

Truman wasn't the first person to suggest the value of owning a dog. The phrase "man's best friend" has been associated with the domesticated dog as far back as the 1700s. I have owned numerous dogs and can honestly say their loyalty is impressive. The only flaw with gaining a dog's loyalty is that the interaction is one-dimensional—your dog is the one who has you on a leash.

Today's longer living male boomer does not live in a one-dimensional world. He lives in an emotionally charged world that demands two-dimensional human-to-human interaction. These unplanned interactions are so unpredictable that most men amusingly refer to them as living in the real world. Our new real-world responsibilities include doing what's best for our spouse, children, parents, and friends—short and long term. The amount of stress behind each of our decisions will depend on each person's health, emotional stability, and financial status, as well as the outcomes of our previous interactions. Keep in mind that by definition every one of us is also going through our own array of physical, mental, and emotional changes.

For example, our typical aging-MBB may have to decide how to handle end-of-life decisions for his father, his mother's diagnosis of Alzheimer's, his spouse's terminal illness, his son's tragic car accident, or his granddaughter's congenital medical condition—while simultaneously having to deal with his own financial and emotional setbacks that accompany his ability to retire. More troublesome is the hidden stress caused by his need to remain calm and in control during any or all of these scenarios.

I have found the most frightening real-world test for the aging-MBB happens when he finds out that he is the one with the terminal medical diagnosis. This scenario requires the additional burden of having to find someone who will take his baton and use it to safely guide those who remain across their ever-changing finish lines.

When faced with any of these real-world scenarios, I doubt the first line of support you would turn to for help and advice would be your dog. I suggest you find someone who understands your perspective, which is another aging male baby boomer—ideally, one who is going through a similar scenario.

I am convinced that finding support from fellow aging-MBBs should be at the top of our list of healthy habits. It is well known that support groups like Alcoholics Anonymous and cancer survivor groups can be an effective way of surviving life's adversities. The support, resources, insight, and tools that are shared by people facing the same battle can make a life-changing difference.

One source that validates my belief that men need each other for support comes from John Gray's successful book, *Men Are from Mars, Women Are from Venus*. Gray doesn't view gender in terms of superiority or abilities but simply chooses to educate the reader that male and female brains are developed differently. His approach to explaining that men and women respond differently to the same event, crisis, or tragedy gives further credibility to why aging-MBBs need to maintain male friendships.

Most men are familiar with the fight-or-flight response. With men, a typical scenario involves a dominant male confronted by a physical stress. He either flees the situation or stands and fights. The option of sitting down and expressing his feelings or sharing his fears is not usually considered as a third option. Conversely, women do not intrinsically share this fight-or-flight hormonal response, which researchers cite as one of the reasons they tend to survive longer than men.

This is why I believe every aging-MBB could actually benefit from adopting a new way of responding in certain situations. Specifically, research shows that both men and women who were able to form strong social ties via marriage, maintain regular contact with close friends, or engage in community organizations had a better overall health status. Support groups can even contribute to better outcomes for men recovering from heart attacks or experiencing heart disease.

You are better off becoming a social creature when dealing with your real-world battles involving health issues, financial struggles, or emotional problems. Remember there are 35 million other MBBs facing similar scenarios. There is no need for any of us to walk this path alone.

Clinical research actually supports the value of helping others. Studies show that people are happier when they give either time or money to those in need. Most importantly, the degrees of happiness don't necessarily correlate with the amount of time spent or money donated, but people are simply happier when given the opportunity to help others improve their lot in life.

Once again, I have gathered relevant personal insights from watching the careers of professional athletes. It has been my experience, after contrasting winners and losers in both team and individual sports, that the main reason male athletes need or benefit from a social connection can be summed up in one word—*accountability*.

All male world-class athletes are clearly driven by the need for competition. These are superstars who choose to fight rather than flee in their arena of performance. Each one chooses to spend years of his life alone training and claims it is the reason he's able to perform at a world-class level.

Ironically, I have found there is only one difference between athletes who set world records and those who simply compete at the world-class level. Those who set world records are willing to allow a coach, teammate, or trainer point out his performance flaws and weaknesses. His openness to constructive criticism is what keeps him accountable—to himself, his teammates, and his training program.

My observation is not a tightly held secret. In fact, it is the main reason why professional teams make the financial commitment to having veteran leadership in their locker rooms. Veteran athletes learned that being a highly competitive, never-back-down loner isn't enough to win championships or set world records. Each knows his success came in part from having a veteran teammate who helped and supported him when he was struggling to achieve any level of success. This realization is also why most veteran athletes find enjoyment in teaching the young, energetic athlete that long-term athletic success is only possible if an athlete is willing to minimize his weaknesses.

This scenario is best shown when a retiring athlete is asked what he will miss most about competition, and he responds, "The connection I had with my teammates." In essence, he's saying his enjoyment and success was due to his teammates helping each other become more successful by holding each other accountable for improving their weaknesses or flaws.

The good news for every aging-MBB is that camaraderie through accountability is not solely reserved for the locker rooms of professional athletes. Accountability does not need a physical location; it only needs an emotional commitment. Military war veterans know this well. They are committed to the simple, yet profound, statement, "Leave no man behind." It was also evident in the early 1900s when American farmers joined together to form threshing crews so everyone could have a successful harvest. Both of these examples demonstrate a man being held accountable for another man's benefit.

Today men gather in church basements, VFW halls, and community centers to share their passions and ideas about improving themselves. They also gather on golf courses, on lakes for long fishing trips, or on the road for Saturday morning bike rides. In these scenarios, at day's end, the majority of men will state the physical outcome of the activity is not the main reason they chose to participate. The truth is, men still find some benefit in being held accountable and remaining socially connected.

My huge caution to the aging-MBB is to differentiate between men who believe, "What happens in Vegas stays in Vegas," to those men who believe the main reason they gather is to help each other become better husbands, fathers, businessmen, and human beings. Always enjoy your favorite gatherings, but do not lose the opportunity to ask for help, advice, or support about topics that really matter. The list includes your inability to quit smoking, challenges in losing weight, reluctance to schedule medical screenings, and troubles rebuilding broken relationships. The ultimate goal is to find a group that values social camaraderie but understands the importance of constantly improving each other.

The great irony is that most aging-MBBs are painfully hesitant to ask for help, yet each finds great joy when given the opportunity to provide help to others. My guess is every one of us has already whispered the words "someday, I would like to be able to provide the same level of help, advice, and support that I was provided when I was struggling." In essence, every male—regardless of the location of his life's locker room—is like the veteran professional athlete who understood the value of helping other teammates become successful.

The wake-up call for the longer-living, aging-MBB is to realize that we—like the professional athlete—will eventually be forced to look back on life and answer the question, "What will I miss the most about my life?" My hope is you will recite the same answer—"The connection I had with my teammates."

I am convinced—it's easy to make new friends, but every aging-MBB has already found out he can't make old friends—he can only choose to maintain them.

I have included space on the www.danielzeman.com website where you can post some of your favorite gathering spots and share the value you have found in maintaining male friendships.

⑦ DON'T TEMPT YOUR APPETITE

Every once in a while, a well-funded and well-designed research study comes along and profoundly states the obvious. My favorite example of such a study found that people buy more groceries if they go shopping when they are hungry. While there is always some benefit in proving the obvious, I wish the researchers would have asked a few other questions such as, "Why do you find food so tempting?" and "Why are you tempted to consume foods or beverages that you once found so unbelievably distasteful?"

As I see it, the answers to these questions would provide every aging-MBB greater insight as to why his emotional temptation can override his biological need for food and beverages.

Everyone has to figure out what triggers our emotional attachment to the food and beverages we consume. I say this because our temptations have clearly changed from our childhood days, when a glass of milk, two Oreo cookies, and a white bread sandwich with bologna and mustard was considered as good as it got.

Today, each of us can easily go into great detail regarding the preferred locations of our favorite dinner meals, casual comfort foods, happy hour hotspots, and specialty café with desserts. Our emotional connection to these gatherings becomes even stronger when we get to choose who is joining us at the table, lounge, or beach-side location.

Food and beverages have always been a cornerstone for all types of social gatherings. America turned the fourth Thursday in November into a national holiday and then created and marketed an entire turkey-themed menu that has survived for generations. Milestone birthdays and career retirements have always involved plenty of food and beverage toasts to the honoree. In addition, guests at these events might even be viewed as disrespectful if they were to say no to the cake.

I find the greatest irony discussing food and beverage consumption in the Christian bible. It defines excessive eating and drinking by the sin of gluttony, yet discusses the celebratory significance of food and wine when it highlights the wedding at Cana. It goes into great detail about the timeline of serving the cheaper wine to the guests and the profound shame of running out of wine at the wedding.

It has been my personal and professional experience that people who struggle with maintaining an ideal healthy-living weight are mentally unable to differentiate between the emotional desire for food and the biological need for calories. For these people, the consumption of food or beverage has become a source of something deeper than basic survival. The question remains: What triggers the emotional connection to food and beverages?

Every aging-MBB needs to understand that food and beverages can trigger both physiological and psychological responses. The psychological responses are linked to our desire to indulge in favorite family recipes or celebrate traditional holidays that trigger strong emotional memories. The physiological responses are usually caused by swings in blood sugar levels caused by skipping meals or eating foods that cause a rapid rise in blood sugar levels.

Finally, most of us were part of the clean plate generation. We ate everything on our plate, no matter the serving size, out of respect for our mother or dinner host and starving children in Biafra (Africa).

Today, most hospitals, weight loss, wellness, and fitness centers promote the message of moderation when it comes to food and beverage consumption. I admit this is a step ahead of their previous message of good and bad foods, but both messages fail to define a measurable number of calories that can be safely consumed throughout the day.

My approach has never changed, and I suggest that every aging-MBB view food as basic fuel, similar to how we view putting gas (fuel) into our car. Without fuel, the car can't take us out on the highway of life. My point is this: food and beverages can be measured and replaced as needed, just like fuel for your car. My goal is to remove the relative terms like *good* and *bad* or *moderation* and arrive at an objective and measurable number of calories.

It is important to remember one basic difference between putting fuel in your car and fuel in your body—that is, your car's gas tank cannot be overfilled. You would never think of trying to pump thirty gallons of gas into a car with a twenty-gallon gas tank. The excess gas would pour out all over the ground at the gas station. But many of us who were introduced to the clean plate club were never told the food we ate was only supposed to refill our empty fuel tank.

Unfortunately, our bodies, unlike our cars, can find room for excess fuel that gets stored in billions of fat cells scattered throughout our bodies, and which leads many of us to rationalize our over-fueling by saying, "That's okay. I can overeat today, because tomorrow I'm going to start exercising."

I believe the key to changing from an emotional temptation about food is to become more objective and simply measure the number of calories we burn off in a day. This doesn't mean we have to completely remove the emotion because you really can't ask Grandma to put a little less love in her home-cooked meals or take away the party from our party foods or worse remove the romance from a romantic dinner.

The simplest way to define the number of calories you burn off in a day is to put calories into two categories. The first category is the number of calories your body needs to stay alive. These include such routine tasks as maintaining your body temperature, muscle mass, bone density, fluid status, and brain function, but muscle mass tends to be the biggest influencer. The sum of each of these expenditures is commonly referred to as your basal metabolic rate (BMR). It can be measured directly using an oxygen consumption analyzer or estimated by using the Revised Harris-Benedict BMR Equation (visit www.danielzeman.com to calculate your BMR).

One example: a sixty-year-old man who is 5 feet 9 inches and weighs 185 pounds would have a BMR of 1,520 calories/day.

The second category is the number of calories your body needs to allow you to move throughout the nonresting parts of your day. This list includes each and every task including bathing, dressing, walking, occupational requirements, hobbies, social gatherings, and, for some people, structured exercise programs. Once again, this number can be directly measured or estimated. Let's assume the guy in our example burns off an additional 480 calories throughout his day.

Using these two pieces of data, our sixty-year-old man burns off 2,000 (1,520 + 480) calories each day. The ability to measure the number of calories he burns off in a day allows him to know how many calories he needs to fill (refill) his body's gas tank—without overfilling it.

The final concerns regarding caloric (fuel) intake are deciding how many times a day our guy should add fuel and how many calories to add at each refueling. The following points highlight the relevant research on refueling times.

- The human brain works best when blood sugar levels are kept consistent throughout the entire day.

- The majority of the population is able to maintain consistent blood sugar levels with three meals and one or two light snacks per day.

In addition, I also suggest that you understand the following basics about calories in and calories out.

- Every calorie (food or beverage) counts toward your total daily intake.

- The actual size of the caloric serving or the amount of food in a serving is much, much smaller than you think. (There is a difference between one serving and going through the serving line once.)

- You will gain fat weight if you consume more calories

than you burn off. The easiest way to gain 10 pounds of fat over the next 10 years is to consume 10 calories more each day than you burn off (10 pounds of fat will show up as two shoe boxes hanging around your waist).

Finally, I created a simple 1-2-3-4 program that will allow you to determine how much and how often to consume the correct amount of food and beverages. My 1-2-3-4 rule of daily caloric consumption is used to represent 10%, 20%, 30%, and 40% of total daily intake.

Specifically

- The 10% is the number of calories for two light snacks.

- The 20% is the number of calories for a morning meal.

- The 30% is the number of calories for a midday meal.

- The 40% is the number of calories for the evening meal.

Using the data from the sixty-year-old man

- His daily snacks should not exceed 200 calories.

- His morning meal should not exceed 400 calories.

- His midday meal should not exceed 600 calories.

- His evening meal should not exceed 800 calories.

My goals with the 1-2-3-4 rules of consumption were to remove the emotion or temptation behind consuming food or beverages and replace them with objective numbers. In this case, the man will retain the option of choosing his meals and snacks, but each will have an objective measure of caloric limits. He will also be encouraged to have consistent feedings (no skipping meals) as this helps maintain blood sugar levels. He is also better equipped to not overeat because he is able to keep his emotional appetite under control.

The good news for every aging-MBB is that your daily caloric budget is not permanent, and it can still be changed. If you want to consume (eat or drink) more calories in a day, you can increase your caloric budget by increasing either your BMR (basal metabolic rate) or your daily levels of any type of physical activity.

The bad news for the aging-MBB is that both resting metabolic rate and levels of daily physical activity will decrease with age. The data are very clear that men lose about 10 percent of their lean body mass every decade. This means if you're still eating the same number of calories that you ate ten years ago, you're overfilling your gas tank and you will get fatter.

The best example of this scenario happened when I ran into two seventy-year-old men at a wedding reception. Bob and Frank had legendary golf teaching careers in Minnesota. I met Frank in the 1970s and Bob in the 1980s and both were avid golfers and ran successful pro shops and teaching clinics at their own golf courses. Immediately after the hugs, hellos, and humorous comments about getting older, attire, and hairstyles, Frank asked me a simple question: "How come we both still play eighteen holes of golf at least three days a week and still eat the same number of calories each day, but we keep getting fatter?"

At first, I hesitated to respond because each had just finished consuming the type of meal that would have equaled the wedding at Cana! But after looking at two happy- and healthy-appearing men who were able to remain physically active for seventy years, I quietly replied, "The first thing you have to remember is neither of you are thirty-five years old, and my guess is it has also been thirty-five years since you last carried your golf bag and walked the entire eighteen holes of the golf course."

They both laughed and said, "You don't need to remind us we are getting older. We switched to driving a golf cart because we don't hit the ball as straight as we did when we were thirty-five, and we got tired of walking all over the golf course to find the golf ball."

The reason I like this example is because each golfer assumed that getting fatter was only caused by overeating. Each had remained active and hadn't changed their intake of calories yet they were still getting fatter. Their only mistake was failing to update their yearly caloric budgets. The last thirty-five years meant each of them had an age-driven loss of muscle mass that meant a decrease in their BMR. Plus, switching from walking the course to driving a golf cart meant losing out on another 300 to 400 calories for each round of golf.

I ended my conversation with Bob and Frank by saying, "Technically you guys are really not overeating, but you are still eating like you are both thirty-five and walking the entire golf course." I closed by saying, "Keep enjoying the game of golf. Just don't spend so much time enjoying the nineteenth hole. Specifically, you need to cut back about 150 calories each day from your consumption or increase your muscle mass by starting a strength training program."

The irony is every aging-MBB already understands the basic concept of creating and sticking to a financial budget. My guess is that each of us has found ourselves in precarious financial situations akin to people who grocery shop when they're hungry. Our emotional appetites may have caused us to spend more money than we've budgeted or saved on cars, family vacations, holiday gifts, anniversary surprises, or anything else that impulsively whets our appetite during a time when we're pressured to pay for kids' college costs, stash some cash in retirement plans, and put a new roof on the house.

We eventually survived the negative balance by immediately updating our financial budget. Our two options meant increasing the amount of money we made or decreasing the amount of money we were spending. The goal was to get back to the budget where we were not accumulating debt because our incomes equaled our budgeted expenses. In other words, we had to find a way to repay the debt.

The wake-up call for every longer-living, aging-MBB is the inability to differentiate between an emotional appetite for food and the biological need for calories that result in an accumulation of a "fat" debt that still needs to be repaid.

Sadly, most aging-MBBs believe their "fat" debt will only impact their physical appearance and not their future finances. We understand the biggest unknown variable in planning our retirement budget is unexpected medical costs (some tied directly back to unhealthy weight)—unplanned surgery, newly diagnosed medical conditions, ongoing long-term pharmaceutical costs as well as the enormous cost of assisted living/housing due to a loss of physical mobility.

The primary goal of any budget is to maintain an objective approach by removing any emotional influences to our decisions. The inability to control our emotions—like an uncontrolled appetite or uncontrolled purchases—can and will drastically affect our financial retirement plans. For every aging-MBB among us, this will come at a time when we really can't afford it.

You're the driver—with or without a golf cart—behind the wheel of your life. You should never lose out on the enjoyment of consuming food and beverages with friends and family at social gatherings. You simply need to update your daily caloric budget with every year of age. You can mathematically plan ahead by knowing what's around the next corner of your life.

I have included a basal metabolic rate calculator and examples of meals/snacks and their matching caloric content on the www.danielzeman.com website.

⑧ GET UP AND BREAK YOUR FAST

I have always been confused as to why so many Americans incorrectly pronounce the word *breakfast*. Specifically, most seem to get confused by the first five letters and incorrectly say "breck" instead of saying "brake." I believe if we began each morning by saying, "It is time for me to get out of bed and go break my fast," we would all have a better understanding of why breakfast is considered the most important meal of the day.

I have to admit, I never understood the importance of eating breakfast so I usually skipped it. In college, my reason was based solely on my desire for extra sleep, which could have been caused by too many late-night outings. Later, after obtaining my first professional job, my decision to skip breakfast was based solely on saving time. I needed to wake up, shower, get dressed, drive to work, park, and be ready to start working before 8:00 a.m. In other words, the thought of missing out on a regular paycheck outweighed the thought of missing out on a possible health benefit. Keep in mind, in those days eating a healthy breakfast meant preparing, consuming, and cleaning up the mess before getting into the car.

Today, the excuse of having no time to prepare a morning meal has become outdated, as times have changed. The frozen food industry created a variety of one-handed breakfast foods that can be microwaved in minutes and eaten with the other hand on the steering wheel. And the fast-food franchises created drive-through food lanes for those who dine on the way to work. Unfortunately, these changes have removed the excuse of time but did nothing to educate us as to why we should eat a healthy, well-balanced breakfast.

Again, the admirable Dr. Breslow is credited as one of the first medical professionals to believe there were hidden health benefits to individuals who started each morning by eating a healthy breakfast. His longitudinal studies were able to show this simple habit was correlated with a patient's long-term health, but he did not attempt to link the possible cause and effect.

Today's medical research continues to believe in a health benefit to eating breakfast or breaking the body's nighttime fast. A 2013 Harvard study found that men between the ages of forty-five and eighty-two who did not eat breakfast had a 27 percent higher risk of heart attack or fatal heart disease. The researchers could not definitively explain the cause for the increased risk but suggested a reason for the correlation. Unfortunately, the ability to demonstrate the direct link was left to a cumulative belief that skipping breakfast puts a strain on the human body, which over time can lead to insulin resistance, high cholesterol, and blood pressure problems.

As for the trouble with the statistics, it really gets down to the inability to control the single variable of not eating breakfast, as well as the influences of other variables like exercise habits, sleep habits, total daily caloric intake, and family history of heart disease.

I suggest you view eating breakfast as a daily habit that keeps you focused on the bigger goal, which is your long-term health and your ability to live independently as long as possible. Keep in mind, as children the majority of baby boomers ate breakfast every morning and never gave it a second thought. A bowl of cereal, right?

Common sense tells me the real health benefits to eating breakfast are achieved via the other healthy habits that are tied to eating breakfast. For example, I have found the ability to get out of bed in the morning and enjoy breakfast is much easier if I am able to get enough sleep, which means better sleep allows me to enjoy eating breakfast. I have also found that limiting the caffeine or alcohol from my evening meal allows me to get a much more restful night's sleep and therefore means I can enjoy eating breakfast.

The same can be said about the number of calories or the size of the evening meal. If I am able to maintain a balanced intake the previous day, then I won't overeat prior to going to bed—leading to a better night's sleep and an enjoyable morning mood for eating breakfast. In other words, my ability to look forward to eating breakfast is clearly influenced by my other daily health habits.

My experience in working with various men over the years has shown me examples of how the timeline of eating a breakfast morning meal is determined by occupations—for example, the professional NBA athlete, the traveling musician, or the hospital nightshift worker. Each of these occupations have schedules that do not allow them to wake up with the morning sun refreshed and ready for a morning meal called breakfast. Another example—when you land after a red-eye flight, should you go to bed when you arrive or eat breakfast? I am convinced if you can control the time of the breakfast meal, then you minimize a myriad of other medical complications.

The idea of adopting a single morning habit like eating breakfast, which has some deeper health benefit, is addressed magnificently by retired Admiral William H. McRaven in his best-selling book, *Make Your Bed: Little Things That Can Change Your Life and Maybe the World.* His book was the result of his amazing and inspirational speech to the 2014 graduating class of the University of Texas.

His basic belief is that if you begin every morning by accomplishing a task, then you can build off that success. Once again, the act of making your bed every morning has no proven relationship to health, longevity, or personal happiness, but it does create a consistent and solid platform for future success.

The bottom line on eating breakfast for us is to get out of bed and start each day by breaking your fast. The aging process has a way of changing our perspective on the value of being alive and the desire to make each day count. Every longer-living, aging-MBB needs to understand he has been given more mornings than any other generation in history. Realize that yesterday is gone, all you can do is get up and make plans for a fresh start and enjoy breaking your fast.

I have found that eating breakfast, sitting down at the table—not wolfing an egg sandwich from a fast-food drive-through at a red light—allows time for planning the day's activities as well as provides time for personal reflection and rededication to the gift of a new day.

Look for a variety of materials and information
about healthy breakfast foods on the
www.danielzeman.com website.

(9) REMEMBER YOUR MEMORY

The human brain is the most complex and the most underappreciated organ in your body. It has an autopilot switch that keeps your heart in a perfect rhythm of continuous flow, a separate sleep mode (although it always stays awake), the ability to recognize distinctively different senses (touch, taste, smell, sight, sound), and the ability to coordinate a three-dimensional athletic movement with such grace that it mimics floating in thin air.

If these aren't impressive enough, your brain also has an unlimited storage capacity for faces and places that can instantaneously create a wide array of raw human emotions (e.g., love, sadness, joy, pain, happiness) that literally make life worth living.

The idea that your aging brain needs to be exercised is a concept that has been totally neglected in today's fitness messages. The fitness industry has clearly identified specific exercises that target the heart, lungs, muscles, and skeletal joints, but the key that drives all human movement or interaction starts in the brain. The most important fact about your brain—like any other muscle or organ inside your body—is that it atrophies with disuse. However, why the brain atrophies should quickly become the number-one concern for the aging-MBB.

In fact, the latest CDC report on brain function should serve as a wake-up call. The results from a survey of almost 60,000 baby boomers showed that one in eight people between the ages of sixty and sixty-four admitted to experiencing increased confusion or memory loss compared to the previous year. One-third of those subjects stated the problems interfered with their work, social activities, or ability to perform household tasks.

Some believe that one possible reason for the brain's inability to maintain its peak form could be a lack of blood flow to the brain. Others believe the decline in brain function could be a long-term cumulative effect of not keeping the brain stimulated with activities such as reading books, doing math problems, engaging in meaningful conversation, or solving simple everyday problems.

One of the most frightening questions for every one of us male boomers concerns how long our brain's hard wiring will last as we continue to live longer and longer.

Each of us grew up believing we could remember anything, like how to ride a bike, sing the lyrics to a song, or play a musical instrument. We were taught, "Once you learn it, you will never forget it." This may actually prove to be true in some cases. A clinically diagnosed Alzheimer's patient can remember the lyrics of a childhood song or still play a musical instrument that he hasn't played for years. Unfortunately, he may no longer be able to identify his spouse or children, though, which we know is an absolutely heartbreaking experience.

I suggest that every aging-MBB consider his brain to be like Siri on his smartphone. When he uses Siri, he is able to engage with a very complex operating system by simply asking questions: "Siri, text Marilyn and ask what I should bring home for dinner," or "Siri, what is the temperature outside?"

In a similar fashion, the human brain is also a very complex operating system that has its own hard-wired connection to every contact that lives within the body. In essence, every task the human body performs was first initiated by the brain's own Siri telling the brain to move, start, find, recall, or maintain some organ of the body. Even more impressive is that the majority of these requests are carried out without our conscious knowledge and yet others while we are sleeping.

I feel this is an important analogy because it allows all future brain research to widen its perspective and show a positive correlation between a healthy brain and the ability to perform all types of social, emotional, and cognitive engagements that may or may not include physical movement.

This wider perspective is extremely important to the aging-MBB because it demonstrates the value of staying socially, emotionally, cognitively, and physically engaged throughout his lifetime. Studies have shown that physically active older adults retain their sense of touch, taste, smell, balance, and memory at higher levels compared to sedentary younger generations. In other words, the aging human brain is still capable of deriving a training effect as long as it stays engaged.

It is safe to say that modern medicine has been slow in conducting research that studies the health benefits of continually stimulating an aging brain. Instead, the medical research model focuses on the diseased or unhealthy brain, because it allows for a clear and definitive medical diagnosis. The good news is that this single-focused approach has successfully provided relief for millions who have been diagnosed with Parkinson's, multiple sclerosis, brain tumors, and strokes.

There has also been ample research on mental illness, including depression and posttraumatic stress disorder (PTSD), often diagnosed in military veterans, police officers, or accident survivors who witnessed unimaginable tragedies firsthand and then were quickly forced back to mainstream life.

To further explain the human brain's wiring, I like using the analogy of turning on a light bulb in a dark room. All of us have walked into a completely dark room and quickly found the electrical switch on the wall. We simply flipped the switch and instantly saw everything in the room.

This example parallels the successful and uninterrupted wiring of the brain of our youth. However, the aging process can cause some delay between flipping on the wall switch and experiencing instant light. As we age, the analogy allows us to determine if our new struggle is finding the switch on the wall, determining if the wall switch is functional, or assessing if the wiring in the ceiling has been interrupted. Going further, we also need to discern if the light socket has become defective or if the light bulb is still capable of turning on with the same brightness we enjoyed in our youth. The human brain remains a highly complex series of electrical connections that is impacted by the aging process.

Here are a few of the real-life hard wiring difficulties we may experience as we age:

- Driving a car: taking more time to step on the gas pedal when the light turns green or to step on the brake when the light turns red; difficulty maintaining a constant speed when driving; the ability to correctly judge the speed of crossing or oncoming drivers; inability to stay in your traffic lane and not swerve back and forth when the wind is blowing.

- Computing simple math/numbers: difficulty adding a 20 percent tip to the total bill after eating at a restaurant or calculating an item's final sale price that includes bonus discounts and taxes; instantly switching from addition to subtraction when balancing your bank account; calculating a person's age from birth years; or recalling phone numbers and house numbers

- Following instructions: challenges with opening a box and correctly assembling all of the parts; navigating through an airport terminal or transit station; or finding your way home (walking or driving) in the dark after visiting a new location

My challenge is to get the aging-MBBs to appreciate the unimaginable complexity of the brain and accept that its current hard wiring may not be as fast or precise as it was in our youth. But accept that such change is part of the aging process.

We must strive to maintain our brain's ability to interpret all of the human senses, maintain speech patterns, recall faces and places, as well as experience raw human emotion—all factors that make life worth living. Sadly, one of our most frustrating times occurs when we struggle to gracefully coordinate any movement patterns that we once took for granted. It is then we will all begin to understand the complexity of the human brain and the importance of remembering to stay actively engaged.

My suggestion for every aging-MBB is to start a two-pronged, body-brain exercise training program that specifically targets the brain.

The first step is to regularly increase highly oxygenated blood flow to the brain by engaging in short bouts of daily physical activity. These exercise breaks are analogous to our elementary school recess, meaning we get up off our chair, shift our focus off what we're doing, and just move. Every human brain cell needs a steady flow of rich, oxygenated blood. The purpose of these breaks is to force your heart to beat faster and your lungs to breathe deeper, which results in a higher percentage of oxygen saturation levels in your brain.

The Mayo Clinic is currently conducting research that demonstrates this concept. Their data show a connection between the deteriorating change in a person's walking gait and declines in memory or thinking abilities. Quite simply, a person's ability to continuously and rhythmically swing opposing arms and legs in a repetitive fashion is tied to their future ability to remember or think.

If you want to see objective proof of the change in blood oxygen levels when moving your body, you can wear a pulse oximeter on your finger and compare the levels before and after the bouts of physical activity. My guess is every aging-MBB who has had a recent medical procedure has probably worn a pulse oximeter during his hospital stay and has witnessed the changes in his own oxygen saturation levels.

In addition to daily physical activity, the next step in the two-pronged brain exercise program involves choosing any activity or task that stimulates a specific part or region of your brain. These are not necessarily physical activities, but they are activities that stimulate the brain. Ideally, you will choose to perform a variety of different tasks each day, or you can choose a different task for each day of the week.

Here are some examples: you can find a new hobby, learn a new language, play a musical instrument, plant a seasonal garden, write a handwritten note, build something, learn to cook, do a crossword puzzle, learn to square dance, volunteer at a charity event, or simply ask a young child if you can help them with their math, science, history, or language homework.

My point is that each of these tasks requires a separate part of the brain to be engaged, which leads to an awakening of those nerve endings. You are turning on the light bulb in that specific area of the brain.

Another way to view the complexity of the brain is to consider each of the tasks just mentioned as if they were different parts of your body that all need to be trained. Considering this analogy, if your goal is to increase your overall level of muscle strength, you would never perform a twelve-week, daily exercise program that requires thirty minutes of nonstop bench presses, because that only challenges one part of your body, which means all of your other muscles would receive no benefit. Similarly, exercising only one specific part of the brain is not a sufficient training program for the entire brain.

It has been my observation that the main reason why most senior citizens become disengaged or withdrawn from society is they stop using those different parts of their brain. In other words, they simply quit turning on the light switches to many parts of their brain. Those once bright and shining areas start dimming down. For most seniors, this process begins innocently. Their confidence begins to erode over time when they engage less of their brain. They eventually become embarrassed when they struggle doing things they perceive as lacking intelligence. Eventually, as this downward spiral continues, they ultimately become less and less engaged with others and feel irrelevant in the fast-paced modern world.

The wake-up call for every aging-MBB is realizing he is responsible for maintaining a healthy and active fully functioning brain. We need to keep turning on the light switches to every part of our brain, not just those in which we have had previous success. By not doing everything possible to maintain a fully functioning brain, we will eventually force someone else to take care of us. In this case, we will never know how difficult we made it on the people around us, and worse, it will become their final memories of us.

The best news for the longer living, aging-MBB is the aging human brain will be the central focus of future medical research. Some researchers believe dementia and Alzheimer's are the greatest health concerns of this century. Their new research will address in-depth questions regarding the aging brain's ability to still learn new tasks, remember new faces or places, and assign an emotional response to each scenario. This new research is the next step in furthering our understanding of the differences in the brains of an infant, child, adolescent, teenager, and adult. This research is timely and valuable, because there will soon be 19 million boomers who are going to be living past their eighty-fifth birthday.

There are people who believe (erroneously in my opinion) we have nothing to fear because the human brain is becoming outdated and will be replaced by some super technological artificial intelligence advancement. Though I admit, Siri seems to know a lot. When you ask Siri, "What is a terrible thing to waste?" she'll answer, "The mind or brain."

The difference between our brains and Siri, though, is that Siri's intelligence is not emotionally capable of actually *understanding* why the brain is such a terrible thing to waste, because she has never won or lost anything. In essence, Siri just recites someone else's programmed data, like sitting on the sidelines and not experiencing life herself.

In my opinion, the best comparison between the human brain and an artificially intelligent Siri is found in Theodore Roosevelt's speech entitled "The Man in the Arena." His speech can be summarized: "The credit does not belong to the critic who only points out why the strong man stumbled, but it belongs to the man in the arena, whose face is marred by dust, sweat and blood, yet continues to battle, who knows great enthusiasm, who spends himself in a worthy cause so that his place shall never be the same as with those cold and timid souls who neither know victory or defeat."

Maintaining a healthy brain will provide every aging-MBB the emotional connection into his own personalized "arena." His brain's ability to provide an emotional recollection of his victories and defeats should be his motivation to continue his final and most sincere "worthy cause" of enjoying the new opportunities offered through the gift of living a longer life than any generation in history.

Every aging-MBB needs to take advantage of his brain's unprecedented ability to store its own self-generated data, because that's what makes it superior to Siri. His brain started storing, interpreting, and processing his unique batch of personal data files beginning with his first heartbeat and is constantly creating and updating the files on his own real-life hard drive. His brain also allows him instant access to the emotional memories behind those historic files when he sees a photo, hears a song, touches a hand, or smells something that reminds him of his past. Conversely, Siri is only able to recite or find someone else's data file because she knows neither victory nor defeat.

Stated more bluntly, your brain is the only piece of living computerized hardware that allows you to passionately describe what truly is a terrible thing to waste—your brain. And that is something we all need to remember.

I have included additional information and links on how to engage the aging brain on the www.danielzeman.com website.

⑩ PLAN A YEARLY EVENT

Jack Nicholson and Morgan Freeman in *The Bucket List* started doing all of their life's missed opportunities (their bucket lists) when each was given a terminal medical diagnosis of less than a year. They instantaneously began cramming in events with the hope of making up for lost time. While this "check it off the list and move on" approach may sometimes work, it doesn't allow enough time to experience life in all its fullness.

Don't wait for a terminal diagnosis. I believe planning annual events can benefit the aging-MBB in many ways. Certainly, every one of us remembers the enjoyment of planning and completing events starting back in our teenage years. Events such as going to a movie, having friends over for a meal, singing along at an outdoor rock concert, or taking a weekend road trip topped those to-do lists. The main goal for each of these events was to enjoy the experience. While many of these events went on to become regular annual traditions, others became the source of legendary humor. However, the nonstop timeline of the aging process has forced every aging-MBB to take a deeper look at the purpose and benefits of planning future events.

I believe there are four distinct reasons every longer-living, aging-MBB achieves long-term health benefits from planning a new and different annual event every year. First, we stay motivated by the challenge of setting a new goal. Second, it encourages us to change our old exercise routine and create a new, more event-specific program. Third, it encourages us to learn a new skill or master a new task. Fourth, it gives us the opportunity to adopt a new point of view that ultimately creates a much deeper personal identity. In other words, the main goal for planning an annual event is to challenge us to continue to find new tasks that require us to stay mentally, physically, and emotionally engaged as we battle the aging process.

There was a time when I would have incorrectly suggested we should plan a yearly event that revolved strictly around an intense fitness activity—for example, running in a hometown marathon or triathlon. However, my years of professional experience have shown me that having a single-focused fitness goal year after year is counterproductive because it leads to increased rates of musculoskeletal injuries or potential chronic medical problems.

It is also difficult to compare long-duration endurance performances from one year to the next. Factors such as weather conditions, acute sickness, or age can dramatically alter our finishing time or force us to drop out of the race, if we didn't get injured during the training. I have also witnessed many of these endurance athletes lose sight of the positive reason why they started exercising and become more concerned as to why they can't stop exercising.

Although I still applaud the discipline of the aging-MBB who has a lengthy history of participating in the same endurance events, I now challenge him to switch it up a little and participate in different events every year. This encourages a more comprehensive training effect. When we train for the same event year after year, we begin to reduce the long-term training effect. Specificity of training means the muscles of our bodies adapt to each specific type of training, which is why it's important to rotate activities that engage all muscle groups. Think about the different muscles used when going for a hike, a fishing trip, a hunting trip, a charity run, canoe-ing, a backpacking adventure, or a yearly bike ride (RAGBRAI is Iowa's great bike ride across the state; or just ride one of the segments).

As an aside, farmers realized a similar drop-off when they planted the same crop every year. Today, farmers rotate agricultural crops on a yearly basis, and their long-term production/performance has remained high. For those endurance athletes who can't understand the farmer analogy, remember those early days of vinyl LP records. Specifically, when the needle would get stuck in a groove and the same song would be constantly repeating itself until somebody finally got up and advanced it to a new song. I can still hear the needle scratching. My point, it's time to listen to a new song, and most of your friends would enjoy hearing you sing a new song too.

The takeaway message, when we're focused on only one activity, is that only certain muscles are trained while others atrophy by not being recruited. Expand your list of activi-ties, which forces all of your muscle groups to be used. For example, consistently rotate programs that encourage you to increase not only your cardiovascular strength but also improve agility, flexibility, and balance.

In other words, the easiest way for us to stay motivated in our life's journey is to observe and compare our footprint to what previous generations of men accomplished across their lifetimes. For example, if you take the time to gain a deeper understanding of the historical timeline of the person who created a historic piece of art, literature, or building site, the more satisfaction you will experience once you find yourself standing in front of any of those masterpieces.

Once again, the main goal of every aging-MBB is to continue to find ways to stay mentally, physically, and emo-tionally engaged as we move through the aging process. Our ability to plan an annual event allows us to accomplish all three of these.

Sadly, today most aging MBBs have inadvertently made the choice to stop being engaged. Worse, they eventually accept a lifestyle of watching television for eight hours every day until it literally becomes their never-ending annual event. This dismal, but all too common, scenario should serve as motivation to every one of us to stay mentally, physically, and emotionally engaged as we battle the aging process.

If possible, find someone or something to help you remain committed to finishing your annual event. The physicians who accomplished the RAAM bike ride I described earlier created a strong social connection that helped them stay focused, and it solidified their memory of the event. They also used the total miles they rode as a simple way to raise $100,000 for the Minneapolis Heart Foundation. To this day, I still can't tell you whose heart(s) received the greatest benefit—the four physicians who rode the event, the countless number of patients who continue to benefit from the ongoing clinical research, or mine. In essence, everyone benefits when someone chooses to stay engaged and it starts with planning a yearly event.

I have included a section on the www.danielzeman.com website that will allow you to post your favorite annual events and share the lessons learned with others.

(11) MONITOR ALCOHOL AND CAFFEINE CONSUMPTION

The belief that sipping a glass of red wine or drinking a cup of black coffee offers some type of health benefit has been debated for many years. The flaw in this philosophical debate is failing to understand the research statistics are based purely on correlations and not on any proven cause-and-effect discoveries.

I introduced Lester Breslow earlier—the lifestyle researcher. He was one of the first researchers to give both of these beverages some research credibility when he began questioning his heathy patients about their daily habits. Dr. Breslow felt comfortable stating that moderate consumption of both beverages was correlated to better health status. The mistake is assuming that these beverages will have the same correlated effect on the health status of all individuals regardless of their body type, family history, or genetic code. In other words, the cross-section of patients in Dr. Breslow's population may not accurately represent the entire US population—or you.

For example, common sense might say that a person's income level is the key factor as to who actually drinks red wine regularly. This in turn begs the question: Is it the consumption of the red wine that improves health, or is better health associated with higher income levels? An even more obvious truth is that many people should never drink, period. The great news is many of these people have found the strength to attend daily closed meetings and say the single best thing they did—today—was to avoid drinking alcohol.

As for the possible health benefits of drinking coffee, most people forget that caffeine is medically classified as a stimulant drug. If coffee were ingested as a pill rather than a beverage, my guess is that people might view reliance on caffeine pills as potentially addictive. Yet, the majority of us believe—rationally or irrationally—the best way to wake up in the morning is to rely on the stimulant effect found in coffee. And now I will add Red Bull and other caffeine-containing drinks.

Another point worth making is the enjoyment found in consuming both coffee and alcohol are learned responses. In other words, unlike sugary beverages that most people immediately like, both coffee and alcohol usually require a longer period of time before a person adapts to the taste.

More importantly, the delay in learning to enjoy the taste of each beverage comes after our bodies obtain some type of satisfying mental and physical side effect from each drug.

I would expect every aging-MBB has his own distinct memory about his first experience with coffee or alcohol. The question remains: Are there proven health benefits to those who choose to consume them? Keep in mind that neither alcohol or caffeine will ever make the RDA's (Recommended Dietary Allowance) list of mandatory daily nutrients.

I always found it amusing when Americans go to great lengths to describe a particular wine's sweetness, body, aroma, taste, aftertaste, and region of origin. This subset of Americans passionately believes red wine consumption should be cherished and its medicinal claims should be written in stone. As for my amusement, the simple fact is the overwhelming majority of Americans still prefer to drink beer, and those who drink wine prefer the cheap stuff.

In 2015, total beer sales represented over half of all alcoholic beverages sold in the US with the top two sellers classified as light beer. It is worth noting that each light beer manufacturer also produced a traditional beer, but those sales were significantly less. In other words, Americans will pay for the alcohol in beer but do not want the extra calories. Plus, the dismal sales of nonalcoholic beer underscore the fact that Americans drink beer for its effect. For those who continue to say they would drink nonalcoholic beer if it tasted better, you simply need to remind them that it probably took time to learn to like the taste of any alcoholic beverage.

I am also amused by the number of coffee connoisseurs in America who can wax eloquently about the ideal aroma, acidity, and temperature of a cup of coffee. Whenever I visit a specialty coffee shop, the barista describes these qualities about one of their greatest tasting coffees, but then asks, "Do you want extra room for cream, sugar, cinnamon, or a two-inch layer of whipped cream?" Seems even the baristas have learned that most Americans do not like the taste of black coffee.

As for the debate of taste versus effect with coffee consumption, 2015 data showed roughly 44% of Americans considered themselves regular coffee drinkers and willingly consumed two to three cups of coffee each day. My guess is the statisticians who arrived at those numbers were sitting in front of a computer screen in a small office, trying to stay awake by drinking coffee. Makes you wonder if the researchers would have come to the same robust, timely conclusion if they were drinking only three cups of water. The fact is coffee (caffeine) consumption is now a socially acceptable beverage that can be consumed any time of the day by almost any age group.

My wake-up call regarding alcohol and coffee consumption came from two personal observations. As a child, I remember watching my grandmother make coffee on her stove in her farm kitchen, or as she called it, "put on a pot of coffee." First, she would fill the coffee pot with well water, scoop out coarsely ground coffee from the large tin can of Folgers and put it in the metal basket, put a raw egg on top of the coffee grounds, then close the lid and wait for the coffee to percolate. I now realize that even Grandma knew she had to find a way to hide the taste of old coffee brewed in well water. As for her family's long-standing traditional choice of using a raw egg to temper the taste, real cream was just too difficult to keep chilled without electricity.

As for alcohol consumption, I recently spent some time in the hill country of east Tennessee and was educated on the fine art of making moonshine. It was there that I was taught a long-standing family recipe for moonshine. Once again, the primary goal of their recipe was to hide the bad taste that resulted from using an outside wood-burning distillery.

Ironically, the moonshine recipe used an apple instead of a raw egg to hide the taste of its final product, but the entire process had the same methodical approach as my grandma's coffee making. Additionally, each beverage also had a family serving tradition. My grandmother only served her legendary coffee in a pink Melmac cup. As for the moonshine, no distinct cup was needed. I was told you drink moonshine straight out of the Mason jar and pass it to the person on your left.

My point in highlighting both long-standing family recipes is that each had a single goal of hiding the bad taste, yet each—my grandma and the folks in east Tennessee—realized that both coffee or alcohol were worth brewing and the only reason to drink either beverage was because of their physiological and psychological effects.

I suggest we take a personal assessment and ask ourselves if there is more to our alcohol or coffee consumption beyond taste. To use an exercise metaphor, does the consumption of either allow us to run toward something that makes us a better human being or away from something that we just don't want to confront?

The following points highlight the potential long-term medical consequences or side effects from consistently drinking the caffeine equivalent of more than three or four cups of coffee per day:

- Coffee consumption can contribute to gastric problems such as acid reflux, heartburn, or diarrhea.

- Coffee consumption can lead to irregular sleep habits that erase the benefits of getting a good night's sleep.

- Coffee consumption can contain hidden calories from sugar, milk, cream, or syrups that minimize the chance of maintaining an ideal body weight.

- Caffeine is a hidden ingredient in many products including decaffeinated coffee. Read the labels on all packaged foods or supplements. This can be especially concerning for those who take prescription medications. Ask your physician whether your alcohol or caffeine consumption affects the dosage or benefits of a new or current medication.

The following points highlight the potential medical and emotional concerns or side effects from those who consistently consume alcoholic beverages:

- Alcohol consumption accounts for nearly one-third of all traffic-related deaths from impaired drivers in the US.

- Alcohol consumption is one of the leading causes of cirrhosis of the liver and cancer of the mouth, throat, esophagus, and colon.

- Alcohol consumption is listed as a contributing factor to many preventable injuries, premature deaths, or suicides.

- Alcohol consumption is listed as a contributing factor to mental health problems, including depression and anxiety.

My consistent answer to every aging-MBB who asks me about caffeine or alcohol is this: There is a reason why there is a coffee shop on every corner, of every street, in every city in America, as well as a reason why prohibition of alcohol did not work.

I continue to believe we have to make our own decision on whether we consume alcohol or caffeine. If yes, then we need to identify the maximal number of beverages we can safely consume. To do this, create your own simple numerical spreadsheet of taste versus effect. Record the exact number(s) of beverages consumed when the taste of drinking coffee or alcohol was able to increase the enjoyment of any social gathering or event. Next, record the exact number(s) of beverages consumed when the physiological or psychological effect of drinking alcohol or coffee made the memory of an event an absolute catastrophe. In essence, accept that you have a measurable limitation when consuming either type of beverage.

Appreciate that the aging process will alter your daily or weekly tolerance for both alcohol and caffeine. For example, if you had a hard time holding your tongue, handling your temper, driving a car, or making financial decisions when you were in your thirties, it's safe to say that consuming the same amount of alcohol or caffeine will not improve your chances of filtering any of these decisions during your later years.

The easiest wake-up call for every aging-MBB is to ask a fellow male boomer about your consumption. My guess is every aging-MBB has seen friends who innocently began making a harmful shift in their taste-versus-effect consumption decision. Do not hesitate to ask a friend, "Do you think I drink too much?"

For those who need a more relevant wake-up call on alcohol or caffeine consumption, marijuana is now legal in many states. I mention this because every aging-MBB realizes the decision to smoke pot was never based on how it tasted.

I have included a variety of materials and contact information about the use and abuse of recreational or prescription drugs on the www.danielzeman.com website.

⑫ HAVE FAITH IN YOUR EXIT STRATEGY

The first time I heard someone mention the need for having an exit strategy was in August 1980. I had recently finished my undergraduate degree in business and was looking to find a real job. Unfortunately for me, 1980 was not the year to find a traditional corporate job in America, so I needed to rethink my future. I contacted a successful chain of athletic clubs in Minneapolis called the Northwest Racquet and Swim Clubs. They had recently picked up on the hottest trend of providing group aerobic exercise dance classes to their members and were debating on adding a strength training room inside their premier club.

Their plan was to create a separate room that would include ten pieces of Nautilus strength training exercise machines. In addition, the room would have constant supervision and require an additional monthly fee to use the equipment. The owners, while optimistic about the new trend of supervised strength training, remained cautious about members paying for something other than tennis, racquetball, or swimming. I tried to comfort them by saying that strength training was just the beginning and that eventually selling fitness memberships, as well as tennis memberships, was going to be the future for athletic clubs. It was then I first heard about the importance of having an exit strategy.

The one owner stated, "Dan, do you know why we built our clubs next to the railroad tracks?" After I offered him no response, he said, "Because every business has to have a planned exit strategy and when tennis or your new fitness markets eventually vanish, the railroads will quickly buy our clubs for storage centers. The railroad company is our exit strategy, and every business has to have a planned exit strategy."

Today, some forty years later, I still recall that conversation because I needed to accept the reality that the fitness industry, like everything else, needs to have a planned exit strategy.

I have to admit the owner's belief that the fitness industry would someday die off made our conversation even more alarming. To me, the archaic railroad industry successfully replaced the pony express, but it certainly would not be alive to save the fitness industry, which I knew was about to become part of every city in America.

I share that story because every aging-MBB needs to understand that we have a financial responsibility and moral obligation to have a planned exit strategy. At first glance, some men might not understand the magnitude or scope of their financial responsibility. You are listed as owner on a variety of financial documents, and upon your death the IRS will demand all taxes to be paid in full.

As for the moral obligation, my guess is we have all heard stories or witnessed scenarios where a man failed to provide his spouse, family, or friends with any formal directives regarding his burial plans, end-of-life decisions, or what to do with all of his stuff. Instead, each man adopted the selfish slogan, "Let someone else figure it out after I am dead and gone." The great news is that an increasing number of men have become more objective about planning ahead for their impending death, which we all know is a 100 percent certainty.

Today, this new trend in planning an exit strategy is found everywhere. Most primary care physicians recommend or require their patients to fill out an advance directive and appoint a healthcare proxy to make decisions if the patient is incapable. Financial planners insist their clients create a retirement plan that includes all future expenses including burial costs and a will to further distribute assets to heirs. I find the best example involves the increasing number of elderly who are choosing to openly discuss how they want their personal items shared or distributed among their survivors. In other words, planning ahead for your certain death is no longer a subject that you can avoid or delay discussing.

I firmly believe every longer-living, aging-MBB should take the time to create his own checklist of what to do, when to do it, and how to handle his expected demise before it happens to him. Once you remove the emotion from the scenario, the actual process is really no different than if you were planning to leave home for a very lengthy vacation. You'd take the time to find somebody who would water the plants, pick up the mail, and watch over the house.

For those aging-MBBs who are quick to defend their decision to forgo creating an exit strategy by saying, "My father or grandfather never filled out any of those forms," let me provide you with some key differences between previous generations of men.

Men in previous generations died in all age groups while the majority of baby boomers will all die after the age of sixty-five. Our grandfathers often died suddenly, with little warning. Today, we are likely to be ill for a long time and be treated by medical staff who will be forced to make decisions to perform both life-saving and life-extending procedures. Previous generations of men were not able to accumulate the amount of stuff nor did they have the same tax or legal ramifications as we do. Most importantly, previous generations of men all knew they were going to die but viewed talking about it as a waste of time. I am convinced we will talk about our exit strategies, and that's what will separate us from how our fathers and grandfathers handled their affairs.

Accept the gift of being born into a timeline in which modern medicine ensures you longevity and in which economic growth provided you the ability to accumulate stuff. But be aware that you have the moral obligation and the financial responsibility to create an exit strategy that will benefit future generations.

I believe each generation of Americans has a responsibility to those who preceded them and to those who will follow them. It is easy to forget that, as a generation, every baby boomer was born into a relatively new country on the world's globe. By definition, each baby boomer has some bloodline connection to those who fought in World War II, or further back to those who created our new country or to those who left other countries in search of the personal freedoms and responsibility promised to every American. It is also easy to forget that the First Amendment to the US Constitution includes the freedom to practice a religious faith.

I mention these key points because every exit strategy, end-of-life decision, living will, and healthcare advance directive, including your preferred type of burial, will be easier for you to discuss if you start off describing your First Amendment choice of having a religious faith.

I ask you to have faith in your exit strategy—as opposed to having confidence—because countless number of people have died to keep the freedom of religious persecution as one of the greatest freedoms provided every American.

I found that practicing a faith can be life-prolonging. For example, if an individual's religion demanded abstinence from alcohol or smoking, then they were healthier because they didn't smoke or drink.

I also believe individuals who have a chosen faith are able to find comfort in times of personal grief or loss. I am continually amazed at the differences between how men of faith deal with the loss of loved ones. Every longer-living, aging-MBB will most likely encounter what the American Bar Association has nicknamed the five Ds: a death, a divorce, a diagnosis, a decline, and another decade. Each of these difficult scenarios will cause him to rethink his exit strategy, and he will find comfort in his personal faith.

The best example of this are the number of Americans who are able to recite the lyrics to numerous gospel songs. The promising lyrics to "Amazing Grace" have made it one of the most recorded songs in music history, and Johnny Cash was quick to share Kris Kristofferson's lyrics that proclaim the possible loneliness of a Sunday morning coming down.

In the end, having confidence or faith in your planned exit strategy will be a matter of personal choice. It will not change your financial responsibility or moral obligation to have a planned exit strategy. Nor will it change the need to update your exit strategy because you are living longer than any generation in US history. My suggestion is to respect those who created the First Amendment and find comfort in their decision to provide you with the right to choose a religious faith, as I believe it will provide you with the confidence to share your planned exit strategy with the next generation of Americans.

I have included information regarding healthcare advance directives on the www.danielzeman.com website.

CHANGE THE COURSE OF THE REST OF YOUR LIFE

These twelve healthier and cleaner dirty dozen habits will not change your mortality, but as Lee Marvin convinced his twelve soldiers, it is possible to change the course of the rest of your life.

In the movie, an eclectic and diverse group of similarly aged men are given a second opportunity to change their life's story. Prior to the movie, each man had made a series of choices that accumulated to the point where each was either sentenced to death or would spend his years confined in a prison cell without the ability to enjoy the everyday freedoms they took for granted. Each man decided this second opportunity on life was too great a gift to pass up. However, it also meant that each man had to totally commit to a structured daily training routine and accept that his commitment would not guarantee him a longer life. His only guarantee was that making the daily commitment would provide him the opportunity to change the ending of the story of his life. In essence, the ability to change his legacy.

I believe the movie's premise is figuratively the same for every one of us aging male baby boomers. Each of us needs to understand that our current stage in life is due to the accumulation of our previous choices and decisions. More importantly, we have the ability to take control of the direction of our long-term health by committing to making better health choices.

While my twelve habits will not completely guarantee a carefree longer life if you follow them, they will reduce the financial burden caused by continuing to make poor health choices. Most importantly, they will increase your chances of living independently and making sure you are able to enjoy the simple everyday freedoms that are almost always taken for granted.

For those who are struggling to find the motivation to change your daily habits, I suggest you consider the lyrics from the Beatles when they asked if you'll still love me when I am sixty-four. But add a new closing verse, "Will you still feed me, will you still bathe me, will you still visit my door when I am eighty-four."

6

NOBILITY—THE SUM OF YOUR FLEXIBILITY, MOBILITY, AND AGILITY

"Do I really need to begin an exercise program?" That's the most common question I get from my fellow aging male boomers.

Here's my answer: "Tell me about your daily habits."

My reasoning is based on the fact that a man cannot erase the negative consequences of his unhealthy habits by simply starting a structured exercise program. In other words, you can't outrun lung cancer; you can't reenergize the life into someone who doesn't get enough sleep; and you'll never shrink the size of a constantly overfed fat cell—the subjects covered in great depth in the previous chapter.

The main reason I wrote this book is to educate my fellow aging male baby boomers (in short, the aging-MBB) that healthy habits create a solid foundation that will allow you to begin to fight the aging process. If your foundation remains solid, then a structured exercise program will provide you additional weapons as you begin your walk across the battlefield that is better known as the aging process.

Your ability to remain mentally and physically active, to stay socially engaged, and to live independently will be determined by how aggressively you battle two very powerful adversaries—aging and automation. The aging process involves a slow but continual deterioration of every cell in your body. Technically, aging can't be defeated, but beginning a structured exercise program is your only legitimate weapon to bring to this battle.

As for automation, I have often said automation is our generation's refined sugar. Both automation and refined sugar were globally introduced and immediately accepted without any concern for their health consequences. Technically, the ongoing acceptance of automated gadgets can't be defeated, but, once again, structured exercise can reduce both the muscle and brain atrophy that accompanies their usage.

Structured exercise programs are defined or classified by their attempt to create a physiological training effect in two major ways:

- A cardiovascular or aerobic program is designed to improve the function of the heart and lungs.

- A strength or weight lifting program is designed to improve the strength or tone of the skeletal muscles.

The simple question for you is which type of exercise program you should do.

The easy answer is both, as cardiovascular and strength exercises have been shown to have significant health benefits. Every aging-MBB needs to understand that we lose 10 percent of our lean body mass (LBM) every year starting at age forty (yes, that hill is not at age thirty but forty, and once there, we are over the hill). Choosing to spend time doing strength training exercises will reduce the loss of muscle mass and maintain your peak strength levels.

You also need to appreciate the fact that heart disease is still the leading cause of death for men. Choosing to spend time doing aerobic exercises will improve heart function and blood lipid levels. However, my suggestion to the longer living, aging-MBBs is to take a deeper look into the negative effects of the aging process before you make an everyday commitment to begin a structured exercise program.

My experience has shown me the deeper answer is found by understanding both the negative effects of the aging process as well as gaining a better understanding of the intrinsic fears found in aging men.

It has been my observation that the majority of aging men (in the fifty-five to seventy-five range) do not fear dying. They are able to remain objective about death and understand it is a natural part of life. However, they clearly have an emotional fear of not dying, especially if they have lost the ability to maintain the intrinsic qualities of what makes them men, which is their masculinity.

I believe today's world of gender-based political correctness incorrectly defines masculinity as arrogance, pride, stubbornness, aggressiveness, ego, conceit, or a desire to remain superior. The medical truth is men are born with a significantly higher level of the hormone testosterone than women, and those higher levels can cause men to demonstrate many of these responses. However, it has been my observation that the emotionally stable aging male really fears losing something that I prefer to call his nobility—not his masculinity.

Examples of these losses tend to start slowly but soon begin to pick up speed. They start when a man notices increasing levels of daily fatigue and a lack of mental alertness. The next progression includes men having difficulties getting up and down stairs, maintaining balance, preparing meals, getting dressed and managing finances. Eventually, men become unable to carry heavy objects, to perform yard work, or to safely drive a car. Next, they choose a walker or a wheelchair for getting around because it's easier than shuffling their feet across the floor.

The final disabling blow to men who choose to ignore the effects of aging and automation is apathy—as these men literally lack the desire to stay engaged with anybody or anything.

I believe every aging-MBB has known or seen many men go through each of these stages. And that is why I can honestly say an emotionally stable man does not fear dying, but he fears becoming helpless and living the final years of his life in a state of total dependence on others to bathe, feed, dress, and get him out of bed every morning.

I realize that some will classify these fears as a man being unstable because he desires to remain superior, prideful, or dominant. My response is to draw a comparison to the aging female's subjective and emotional approach to her death. It has been my observation that the emotionally balanced aging female—similar to the aging male—does not fear dying.

The statistical truth is women have longer life expectancies than men. They have also watched their mothers and grandmothers remain socially active in spite of their dependency on wheelchairs or being forced to live in assisted care centers. However, this does not mean women do not have their own gender-intrinsic emotional fear about dying.

In 1992, I was asked to volunteer at a 5k walk/run event for a women's health issue. At the time, I was hesitant to volunteer for the event because it was going to be held outside on Mother's Day morning in Minneapolis. I couldn't imagine the event being a success. Why would women get up early and go for a walk, in cold temperatures on the day when they were going to be recognized for their intrinsic gift of being able to be mothers. My other hesitation was the leading cause of death for women in 1992 was—and still remains—heart disease. The medical fact is women were much more likely to die from having a heart condition than the health concern I was volunteering to support.

The statistical truth is women have longer life expectancies than men.

The idea behind using organized walk/run events as a method of promoting awareness and increasing the rates of preventive testing and monitoring of a medical condition had become common in Minnesota and elsewhere, but expecting women to get up early in the morning, in cold weather, on Mother's Day just seemed to be a huge gamble.

Today, some twenty-five years later, that Mother's Day walk in Minneapolis continues to draw crowds of 30,000 people and is called The Race for the Cure, and its single goal is to promote research on, educate women about, and eradicate breast cancer. I have often wondered if 30,000 people in Minneapolis would get up on Mother's Day and walk for lung cancer or colon cancer or heart disease. In other words, what is it about breast cancer that brings out the passion and purpose in 30,000 people on Mother's Day?

My point is both men and women do not objectively fear dying. Yet they both become very passionate and emotional about how they prefer not to die. In essence, they both want to hold onto their intrinsic gender identities of being masculine or feminine. The great news for women is their passion for fighting breast cancer has saved lives.

It is my suggestion that every longer-living, aging-MBB accepts that it is okay to fear losing his intrinsic gender identity as a male. I believe his intrinsic fear of maintaining a high function or quality of life is not based on arrogance, pride, or male ego. The idea of being kept alive, yet totally dependent on others, is a scenario that gets to the core of every male. For those who want a proven example of my belief, take a look at the terminally ill cancer patient. The concept of hospice remains the single greatest example of bravery and compassion—regardless of gender—for those trying to accept their impending death. Each patient decides that a life is meant to be lived and not kept alive.

The great news is you can delay the physical effects of aging and ensure you are able to maintain your nobility. You simply need to begin an exercise program that allows you to retain your flexibility, mobility, and agility.

WHY FLEXIBILITY?

Imagine having the ability to smoothly move every skeletal joint through a complete range of motion without limitations? That's my definition of flexibility. Getting up off the floor after playing with grandchildren would be much easier, and so would cleaning the garage or mowing the lawn.

The importance of maintaining your flexibility is often forgotten in today's exercise culture that prefers to promote high-intensity exercise programs. These programs are designed to deliver immediate results with no concern for long-term exercise adherence. But at this stage of life, our goal is to prepare for the next decades of life.

But at this stage of life, our goal is to prepare for the next decades of life.

I recently asked Andre Deloya, a longtime friend and one of the most talented physical therapists in the country, to answer this question: What is the single greatest advice you would give today's aging male baby boomer?

He thought about it and then without interruption said, "I would tell him to maintain his posture."

I asked him to explain his statement. Andre shared with me countless stories about the number of patients who mistakenly believe their specific joint pain is only related to that joint. In other words, most fail to recognize their knee pain is actually caused by having poor ankle joint mechanics, or their right hip pain is actually the result of them compensating for their left knee mechanics or their neck pain is being triggered by their shoulder positioning.

My guess is every one of us who has seen a physical therapist for any type of rehabilitation will remember being told something like "before I work on your knee, I will need to check out your hip." The key takeaway is your ability to move a particular joint through a complete range of motion without any limitations is really based on the flexibility of the other joints of your body.

Most men who find themselves struggling with pain or a lack of motion in a specific joint will overcompensate by changing their movement pattern. Big mistake. The simplest example: you feel as if you might have a rock in your shoe, so instead of stopping and removing the rock, you continue walking but choose to adjust your walking gait so the rock doesn't cause pain.

This scenario is easily expanded to include individuals who develop neck pain caused by spending a lot of time in front of a computer screen. They eventually find difficulty with lifting their neck up to see the top of the screen, so instead of stretching their neck, they choose to buy a different chair. The same is true for people who begin to struggle putting on a shirt because of difficulty lifting their arms above their heads. They soon find another way to put on their shirt, or, worse, they buy a different style of shirt.

My point is that, when we begin to lose flexibility of one joint, we are actually putting additional stress on other joints and eventually limiting the range of motion of those joints.

The takeaway for us is to realize our ability to enjoy a high quality of life with a high level of function will be based on our ability to maintain or improve our levels of joint flexibility. We live in a three-dimensional world, and our bodies were designed to bend, twist, or rotate in all three of those dimensions.

We live in a three-dimensional world, and our bodies were designed to bend, twist, or rotate in all three of those dimensions.

The main reason to increase your flexibility is it will allow you to move freely across the entire range of motion of your youth. Once you begin to lose your body's normal range of motion, you begin to shorten the range of motion of the world around you.

WHY MOBILITY?

The main reason to maintain your mobility is to allow you to move smoothly or freely across the entire range of motion without hesitation or interruption.

The reason why we fail to appreciate our mobility is that we no longer move our body in all three dimensions. The majority of our movements have become reduced to a single plane—that being a forward motion. The loss of three-dimensional movement only increases the rate of atrophy to the muscles that are no longer being used. In other words, today's aging-MBB no longer moves sideways, walks backward, or stands tall.

Additionally, the aging process is continually accelerating the rate of muscle atrophy regardless of our levels of movement. This will result in an ongoing loss of muscle strength. The loss of strength includes both a muscle's ability to lift and lower a weight—more commonly referred to as concentric and eccentric muscle contractions in my world.

The best example of this loss is what I call a flopper. I have known many floppers, and they all started out innocently and uninformed by choosing to take the escalators instead of walking up and down the stairs. They failed to understand that walking up the stairs engaged their quadriceps muscles in their frontal thighs by lifting their body weight via a concentric contraction. More importantly, walking down the stairs involved using the same thigh muscles to lower their body weight via an eccentric contraction. Eventually the use of the escalator became the preferred mode for getting up and down stairs. Unfortunately, it also meant a loss of concentric and eccentric strength in the quadriceps muscles.

As for why I call them floppers? Picture a man who lowers himself down onto his favorite corner of the couch or into his recliner. He begins by backing up to the couch and then slowly lowering his body weight via an eccentric muscle contraction. Eventually those lowering muscles atrophy and lack the necessary amount of eccentric strength to completely lower this dude onto the couch, so instead he simply flops down onto it with a thud.

On a more serious note, the loss of eccentric quadriceps strength is the reason why most men are mistakenly encouraged to use the handrail when walking down the stairs of their homes. Unfortunately, most men believe the need to use the handrail is based on the correlation between falling down the stairs and a lack of balance. I believe a man's inability to slowly and safely use the stairs is often due to his lack of concentric and eccentric strength.

I have heard many men say, "I fell going down the stairs because I lost my balance," but in reality, he resorted to his flopping technique because he no longer had the eccentric strength to lower his body weight.

Eventually, all couch floppers will lose their concentric muscle strength and end up needing assistance getting up from the couch, which has grown an entire business that manufactures lift chairs. As an aside, I have yet to hear any of them say the reason they can't stand up was due to a loss of balance.

The great news is that the human brain and skeletal muscles are capable of regaining the strength that was lost due to aging, automation (escalators), and flopping. The healthy brain is still able to locate the nerves that recruit the specific skeletal muscles, and the muscles are still able to respond to strength-training exercise programs.

The key to designing a strength-training program that increases mobility is to understand the training effect derived from encouraging a repetitive neuromuscular recruitment pattern against a known level of resistance.

The simplest explanation involves the concept referred to as specificity of training. In essence, practice makes perfect. If you want to increase the amount of weight you can lift on a chest press machine, then practice on that machine, using the same grip and the same seat position. Your brain will decide which muscles or recruitment pattern will deliver the best results. While this intrinsic relationship between your brain and muscles is impressive, it is important to realize if you switched chest press machines, your new and improved levels of strength will not transfer. Again, your specific strength training effect was your body becoming better at doing the exact movement pattern you practiced.

The important takeaway is to spend time improving your levels of strength across movement patterns that simulate your daily routine. These simulated movement patterns are referred to as functional strength training, and they are geared toward improving your ability to move freely in multiple planes. They are unique because each movement engages muscles that are specific to the pattern (called prime movers), others that offer assistance (called assist muscles), and finally those that keep the body upright (called stabilizers).

Examples of these include lifting and lowering objects from ground level to over your head, walking and rotating your body's center of gravity, and performing an upper or lower body movement while keeping your abdominals and low back muscles engaged.

I have included easy-to-follow exercises you can do to maintain your mobility on the www.danielzeman.com website.

WHY AGILITY?

Can you respond quickly and safely to unplanned scenarios like falling objects, busy crosswalks, excited children, and anything that suddenly appears underfoot? The aging process not only slows down our brain's ability to remain on high alert, but prolonged inactivity slows down our neuromuscular recruitment patterns that keep us upright.

So I define agility as the ability to react quickly and safely to an unplanned event without suffering unnecessary injuries or harm. Catching that falling can of soup, safely stumbling over the dog without falling, and grabbing a grandchild's hand before she darts into traffic.

If you asked the majority of Americans who among us needs to have great agility, most would respond that athletes do. While this is true, every aging-MBB also needs to maintain his agility. He will no longer be asked to catch the game-winning pass or throw the final strike, but he will be asked to react quickly and safely to a variety of real-life scenarios.

I suggest you expand your definition of mental alertness from a single-focus response to a multi-responsive interactive experience. I believe the bar for mental alertness should be viewed as your ability to mentally and physically respond to an unplanned stimulus—which is ultimately determined by your level of agility.

For example, in our youth, it was easy to walk down the sidewalk carrying a bag in one arm and a cold beverage in the other, plus avoid stepping in a puddle of water without changing stride lengths or spilling the beverage. In other words, our younger body and brain could multitask without causing an overload. Once again, aging, automation, and muscle atrophy due to disuse are the new reasons we need to spend time maintaining our agility.

For those skeptics who believe encouraging longer-living, aging-MBBs to improve their level of agility will only increase their risk of falls and should be avoided, my response is to remind them that the original treatment for patients who had a heart attack was weeks of complete bed rest. Skeptics believed encouraging cardiac patients to walk would only increase the risk of their having another heart attack. This overly cautious approach led to further atrophy and in most cases another heart attack. Today, the accepted rehab for surgical heart patients is to get them standing and/or walking within twenty-four hours of their procedure. The new goal is to avoid having another event by increasing heart function.

I believe that same proactive approach should be used when it comes to decreasing the risks of falling. The new goal is to increase levels of agility, which will keep us mentally alert, as well as maintain our ability to react to unplanned events that would have previously led to a fall or injury.

In summary, the key insight for every aging-MBB who is trying to maintain his nobility is to understand that his brain and his muscles need to work together to successfully orchestrate and perform every daily task.

MOVEMENT IS LIKE A JUKEBOX

The best analogy of task-specific, brain-to-muscle interaction is found in every small-town café or honky-tonk in America that still has a coin-operated jukebox. I have fond memories of dropping in a quarter and pushing the buttons marked B12, G4, and D5. My desired task—wanting to hear specific songs—meant I had to push the correct button that would trigger the jukebox to perform the three-dimensional task of grab, twist, and play the small vinyl 45 for the specific songs in the order I requested.

I also remember that every jukebox had a mandatory list of classic songs like Elvis Presley singing "Hound Dog," Patsy Cline singing "Crazy," and Bing Crosby's "White Christmas." In a similar scenario, every aging-MBB has a list of mandatory tasks that will ensure his nobility—the combination of flexibility, agility, and mobility. His mandatory list of classic tasks will need to include standup and walk, turn around and lift me up, and drop but don't flop. He simply needs to push the correct button and his brain and muscles will perform each of his classic tasks.

I used to wonder why there were so many different types of songs on a small-town beer joint's jukebox. I now consider that variety or number of songs to be as impressive as the endless number of orchestrated movement patterns that can be performed by the human body. In essence, both the jukebox and the human body have a lengthy list of songs or movements that allow them to show off their ability to remain finely tuned and ready to play anywhere and anytime of the day.

However, both are governed by one simple rule: if nobody pushes G10, then that song or that specific task is removed from the list of options. In other words, we can't complain about not being able to find "Walk backward and don't fall down" on our personalized task jukebox when we haven't pushed that button in the last ten years.

In the end, nobility or quality of life will come down to a matter of personal choice. Every one of us needs to decide which tasks or buttons we want to be able to keep pushing. We can decide whether we want our brain to remain on high alert and ready to react. We decide whether our muscles have enough concentric and eccentric strength so our joints can move pain-free through the entire range of motion.

In the end, nobility or quality of life will come down to a matter of personal choice.

We understand that aging, automation, and disuse will slowly remove tasks from our personalized playlist unless we choose to continue to practice performing each task. We also realize our ability to live independently will eventually be determined by our ability to perform simple everyday tasks such as personal hygiene care and basic house maintenance.

In spite of this knowledge, I still believe most men will choose to wait to begin a functional exercise program—that improves their flexibility, mobility, and agility—until the day when they are unable to perform a classic daily task.

If you have a friend who has suffered a stroke, sadly, that's the best motivation or wake-up call we might need to understand the tragedy of loss of nobility. This catastrophic medical event will change our friends from having a full and interactive brain to struggling to find the button on their jukebox. This scenario is one that plays out every day in hospitals and emergency rooms across the US. A physician will ask a patient who has suffered a stroke to move his toes or fingers, and the patient will stare at his limbs in a state of disbelief because he literally cannot find the button that plays that song.

My point is this: Do not delay your decision to choose to push every button on your jukebox. If you begin to struggle to perform any daily task, take it as an early warning sign of an upcoming functional loss. If you choose to ignore a loss of your flexibility, a loss of your mobility, or a loss of your agility, then you will certainly begin to notice a loss of your nobility.

My hope is that men will follow the example that women of every age used to fight against breast cancer. Men of all ages need to become more passionate about losing their nobility. If men are able to look past the discipline and drudgery of structured exercise and see the real goal, then I see no reason why 30,000 men could not jump up out of bed on Father's Day and walk for ALS (Lou Gehrig's disease) or for their friends who had strokes. On that day, it will be clear to everyone in attendance that standing up and fighting for your nobility is a worthy cause.

7

HEART STILL MATTERS

"What's my destiny, Mama?" is one of the memorable questions Tom Hanks asks his dying mother in his Oscar-winning performance in the movie *Forrest Gump*. He also says, "I had run for three years, two months, fourteen days, and sixteen hours." When asked why, he said, "I just felt like running," and humorously shared that "when I got tired I slept, when I got hungry I ate, when I had to go, yah know, I went."

Later he said, "My mama always told me you have to put your past behind you" and "that is why I did all of that running." And here's my point: When he was questioned about the reason he stopped running, he matter-of-factly said, "I'm pretty tired, I think I'll go home now…and just like that my running days was over."

As a baby boomer, I enjoyed the movie because it provided a detailed and reflective timeline of the baby boomers' quirky place in history. More importantly, as an exercise physiologist, I loved the movie because it not only provided a timeline of the running movement, but also posed and answered two key exercise questions: Why do people engage in cardiovascular exercise? And when is it time to stop running?

Forrest Gump was not the first character to discover that long distance running offered some emotional relief or that running was a legitimate measure of athletic performance. The 1896 Olympic Games in Athens, Greece, featured running as one of the ultimate feats of human performance. Olympic officials understood that a runner's ability to win a gold medal was dependent upon the distance of the race, which is why they had separate races for sprinters, middle distance, and marathon runners. Each runner was uniquely gifted in running a specific distance. In other words, a runner could win a gold medal in the sprints but could fail to finish if asked to run a marathon.

Early American marathon runners were also drawn to the allure of running competitions. The first Boston marathon was held in 1897. However, it is safe to say that it took the 1974 invention and marketing of the first legitimate running shoe, the NIKE waffle trainer, before running became a national movement. Yes, the waffle trainer was literally made on a waffle iron and sold like hotcakes.

The biggest advancement in the credibility of the running movement came in 1968 when Ken Cooper coined the word aerobics. Dr. Cooper showed that running and other forms of physical activity that encouraged a continuous pattern of rhythmic and repetitive movement were beneficial to the heart and an effective way to reduce stress. You could say running was proven to be good for your heart, and if you were wearing the right shoes, it was also easy on your "soles."

The human heart is a uniquely designed muscle with four interactive chambers. These four chambers maintain a continuous symbiotic rhythm of contracting and relaxing—emptying and filling—via an electrical impulse controlled by the brain. The heart is in constant communication with the brain and receives two basic commands: to beat faster/slower and to eject more/less blood per beat. The heart's ability to deliver oxygen to all parts of the body is also influenced by the health status of the red blood cells and the elasticity of the lungs, arteries, and veins.

The heart is in constant communication with the brain and receives two basic commands: to beat faster/slower and to eject more/less blood per beat.

The goal of aerobic exercise can best be described as the heart's ability to deliver oxygen to the exercising muscles. If the heart is able to deliver the optimal amount of oxygen required by the working muscles, then a steady state flow is achieved. Science has also shown that the demand for oxygen rises linearly with work rate. In other words, as you increase running speed, your heart has to deliver more oxygen to your leg muscles.

HOW MUCH IS ENOUGH?

This blood-pumping scenario plays out daily in every health club and is the driving force behind the question: How fast should my heart beat when I am doing cardiovascular exercise?

Initially, this question was answered using a generalized approach that involved observation of the exercising human heart. This big picture perspective started with the assumption that every individual's maximal heart rate was found by subtracting his age from 220. For example, a forty-year-old male was capable of increasing his heart rate to a maximal rate of 180 beats per minute (bpm): (220 - 40 = 180 bpm).

The next challenge involved defining the percentage of a person's maximal heart rate that would elicit a training effect. Trial and error eventually led to the generic recommendation that when exercising, an individual's ideal training heart rate range should be 60 to 75 percent of his predicted maximal heart rate. For example, our forty-year-old with the theoretical max heart rate of 180 bpm was told to exercise between 108 and 135 bpm.

The final variable was defining the ideal amount of time an individual should spend exercising. Once again, trial and error eventually led to the recommendation that the ideal duration should be between thirty and forty-five minutes per session.

This generalized approach to answering the ideal heart rate question quickly became the suggested recommendation to the American public. It also opened the door for the successful invention, marketing, and sales of wearable heart rate monitors. And similar to the success of the early running shoe, heart rate monitoring devices sprinted off the shelves of many retail stores.

However, the biggest assumption made by the fitness, medical, and wellness industries in the early days was believing everyone would enjoy aerobic or endurance exercise. This assumption was in part based on those distance runners who thoroughly enjoyed the quiet solitude of running. Unfortunately, the overwhelming majority of exercisers found endurance exercise to be very boring. So the biggest decision was not whether someone should adopt a regular habit of endurance exercise, but to decide on how he was going to endure endurance exercise.

Once again, technology quickly ran to the rescue of the bored endurance exerciser when the bulky but effective SONY Walkman was created. Today, man and machine both run to a similar beat, as the exerciser shows no sign of turning down the volume when exercising, and manufacturers show no sign of turning down the volume in the number of new products they invent.

Someday, my friends, my fellow aging male baby boomers, your heart will literally stop beating. And just before that moment, you will undoubtedly look back on the times (minutes, days, weeks, years) of your life with fondness or regret. In essence, did you devote too much time doing tasks that proved to be meaningless at the expense of spending time with things that really mattered?

While it is easy to agree with medical science that demonstrates the benefits of aerobic exercise, it's more important to understand the science behind aerobic exercise programs. Specifically, what is the recommended intensity, frequency, and duration of aerobic exercise needed to obtain and maintain a healthy heart?

My reason for encouraging each aging-MBB to understand the difference among these three variables is based on personal experience. I see countless twenty-five to forty-year-old men forcing themselves to endure high-intensity aerobic exercise. They discovered that exercising at higher heart rates also equates to a higher total caloric expenditure. Their single focus is to burn off all the "unhealthy" calories they consumed over the previous weekend. In essence, they are not interested in a program that promotes long-term adherence via moderate intensity, frequency, and duration because they want to burn off as many calories as possible and plan ahead for next weekend's round of beers watching the big game with nachos, burgers, and chip dip.

Conversely, I have also seen a new trend for men in the age range of fifty-five to seventy-five. They have begun to perceive high-intensity long-duration endurance exercise as equivalent to a caged rodent running aimlessly on a hamster wheel. Seems every man eventually realizes that he can no longer view his exhaustive exercise program as heart healthy, nor can he justify taking time away from things that should matter to him.

Seems every man eventually realizes that he can no longer view his exhaustive exercise program as heart healthy, nor can he justify taking time away from things that should matter to him.

In *Forrest Gump*, Tom Hanks's character was able to find a similar wake-up call or aha moment. Gump would eventually decide he was tired of wasting time enduring nonstop endurance exercise without any human interaction and realized it was time to go home and spend time doing what mattered to him.

From an exercise physiology perspective, Gump participated in a three-and-a-half-year aerobic exercise program that clearly prioritized the duration and frequency of aerobic exercise over the intensity. From a philosophical perspective, you could say Forrest Gump found his answer to Bob Dylan's 1963 question, "How many roads must a man walk down before you call him a man?" Every longer-living, aging-MBB who continues to prioritize duration, like Forrest

Gump—the time he spends doing his aerobic exercise program—over frequency and intensity will end up losing out on events that really matter in his life. You could say his remaining years will literally be blowing in the wind.

I have tested the cardiovascular fitness levels of countless individuals. The goal has always been to design an individualized exercise program that guarantees an improvement in a person's cardiovascular fitness level. In essence, my goal is to train people to run down as many roads as possible, as fast as they can without wasting their time.

Each fitness test begins and ends with gathering as much data as possible. The list includes heart rate, breathing rate, a relative sense of perceived exertion, as well as the continuous levels of oxygen consumption and carbon dioxide production. A typical fitness test uses a Graded Exercise Test (GXT) protocol that includes a warm-up stage, a period of increasing workloads, and a recovery stage. The warm-up stage is generally a three-minute effort with an easy level of exertion while on a treadmill or stationary bike where I can control the speed. This is followed by methodically increasing efforts of work until the person becomes exhausted or is unable to continue. The recovery stage is a mandatory cool-down period using a workload similar to the one used during the initial warm-up stage.

My personal takeaway is that all test subjects have similar responses to the three stages of the GXT. They all look refreshed and ready to go during the warm-up phase, but everyone eventually reaches a maximal effort and struggles in the recovery phase. A person's ability to endure more stages during the GXT is based on three variables. Specifically, his heart's current level of function, the mitochondria density within his skeletal muscles, and his ability to tolerate increasing levels of fatigue. These three variables can be improved with aerobic exercise. Keep in mind that eventually a subject's age will become a limiting factor because each of these three variables will lose their adaptability in the presence of aging.

IS THE OUTCOME WORTH THE EFFORT?

I collected the following GXT data on a fifty-year-old named Matthew. Matthew was a well-conditioned male with a twenty-year history of running four to five days per week. He was worried about getting overly fatigued, reoccurring knee pain, and wasting his time doing excessive amounts of cardiovascular exercise. The GXT was performed on a stationary bicycle ergometer with Matthew wearing a VO_2 (oxygen consumption) face mask.

Matthew's key fitness test results were as follows: his maximal aerobic fitness level or VO2 was 44.1 ml/kg/min; his maximal workload on the stationary bike was 280 watts; and his maximal heart rate was 169 bpm. His caloric expenditures increased linearly from 6 kcals to 18 kcals as the bike workload increased from 100 to 280 watts. These measurable results allowed me to create an individualized aerobic exercise for Matthew based on his current level of cardiovascular fitness. I can be very specific with regard to his ideal intensity, frequency, and duration of exercise.

I believe the biggest mistake most people make when designing an aerobic exercise program is believing heart rate is the key variable. The problem with using the heart rate data gathered during any GXT is there are no obvious thresholds, because the slope or increase in beats is linear with the workload. In other words, heart rate data are not capable of defining an ideal training program, because they do not provide a deflection point or threshold to define an ideal training intensity. Additionally, since a person's heart rate will decrease as their level of fitness increases, it is best to design an aerobic exercise program around a variable that doesn't change and can be used as consistent benchmark.

My extensive experience has allowed me to find two other measurements that do provide deflection points or thresholds and are all easily gathered during a GXT. The first considers what is going on inside the subject's brain (mental state) and is measured using the BORG scale or rating of perceived exertion (RPE). The second considers what is going on inside the body and is measured by the total volume of air being exhaled or Ventilatory Threshold (VT).

Once again, the biggest advantage to using either of these variables is that each threshold is associated with a specific workload. This would provide me with a benchmark to create an individualized aerobic exercise program for Matthew that includes a specific intensity, frequency, and duration.

The BORG scale or rating of perceived exertion (RPE) is based on the test subject's collection of physical and emotional sensations felt during the entire GXT. The subject is asked at the end of each stage of the GXT to point to a number on the BORG scale that represents his overall sense of perceived exertion. You might see these charts in your own fitness center.

The original design for using a numerical scale of 6 to 20 was based on an early belief about young test subjects' heart rate responses during a GXT. The hope was that all test subjects would numerically match their BORG score to their heart rate. For example, a BORG 6 would match a heart rate of 60 bpm, a BORG 10 would match a heart rate of 100 bpm, a BORG 14 would match a heart rate of 140 bpm, a BORG 18 would match a heart rate of 180 bpm. In essence, a test subject's perception of exertion would follow the same linear slope of their heart rate throughout the GXT.

Unfortunately, I have never found a test subject's heart rate data to mirror his BORG ratings. The simple reason is the majority of test subjects' perception of fatigue is not linear with their level of effort when riding the testing bike.

As expected, I found that Matthew's BORG ratings were not linear across the twelve stages of his GXT on the stationary bike. His BORG ratings across the first seven stages were relatively similar, yet he was aware the workload and his heart rates were increasing. Things changed at the end of the eighth stage when

Matthew quickly pointed to 15 on the chart and perceived his effort as hard. His BORG ratings continued to increase over the next four stages until he found himself in a state of complete exhaustion.

This relatively simple test allowed me to gather my first insight into Matthew's ability to tolerate aerobic exercise on a stationary bike. It was obvious that workloads above 200 watts would not be attainable or sustainable.

The second variable that I needed to use to create Matthew's aerobic exercise program involved his Ventilatory Threshold. Let me start off with a brief explanation of how the lungs or a person's breathing provide additional insight into creating an aerobic exercise program.

People tell me they want to have a fitness test or start an exercise program because, most often, they recently had an experience where some previous level of everyday physical activity left them winded or feeling like they were sucking air. The physiological reason or cause for these complaints is either a decrease in their maximal level of cardiovascular endurance or an inability to tolerate the same relative intensity of their maximal level of cardiovascular endurance.

What hasn't changed is the basic physiology that says the demand for oxygen consumption (via inhaling) is linear with work, while the production of carbon dioxide (via exhaling) is exponential in the presence of increased levels of work. In essence, when a person complains of breathlessness during intense endurance exercise, it is because they can't stop exhaling, not because they can't stop inhaling.

I have found this exponential change in exhaling to be very audible inside the quiet testing lab. Again, this very audible sound in the testing lab is not from the subject actively trying to inhale oxygen; rather, it is his inability to control or override the body's need to exhale its high levels of carbon dioxide.

The two key takeaways for Matthew were his ventilation, like his BORG ratings, was not linear across all thirteen stages of his

GXT. Once again, his body began to struggle after stage seven or 180 watts. In this case, after 180 watts he was beginning to accumulate metabolic "fatigue" after he completed riding the stage at 180 watts. The only way for him to get rid of his increasing levels of fatigue was to forcefully exhale.

As an aside, the ability to measure the point where exhaling becomes exponential is one of the key reasons world-class endurance athletes prefer to compete without any type of external audio distraction. Greg LeMond refused to communicate with his team car during the final day time trial of the 1989 Tour de France. Greg knew his only goal was to ride the entire distance as fast as he could without having to slow down. The only way for him to do that was to block out any external interruptions and internally focus on his breathing or ventilation.

The good news for us aging-MBBs is that our ability to define our own performance redline can be approximated by using our speech patterns or the ability to talk. I encourage all test subjects to create their own unique ten- to twelve-word sentence and to recite it periodically throughout the duration of the exercise program. If you begin to alter your speech or sentence pattern, then you should quickly reduce the workload.

The good news for us aging-MBBs is that our ability to define our own performance redline can be approximated by using our speech patterns or the ability to talk.

For example, try repeating the sentence, "The older I get, the more I really like classic country music." You will find this sentence can initially be stated without any interruption but will become two sentences when your ventilation rate changes. Specifically, this relatively simple flowing sentence will have a noticeable point of separation where it will become "the older I get...the more I really like classic country music." For those who do not like classic country music, you can create your own mantra—preferably one that is easy to remember.

Although the BORG and the ventilation data do provide an ideal starting workload or intensity of aerobic exercise, neither provides a legitimate answer to the appropriate frequency or duration for the aerobic exercise program.

It took me decades to figure out the connection among these three key variables, and I wish it was more complicated. I have found that choosing the ideal duration (number of minutes) and frequency (number of days/week) are dependent upon the test subject's maximal level of cardiovascular fitness. In other words, subjects with higher levels of maximal aerobic fitness are intrinsically able to endure exercising at the same relative intensity for more minutes a day across more days of the week.

BACK TO HOW MUCH IS ENOUGH?

I created an easy-to-remember template that matches a person's level of fitness with ideal training durations and frequencies. Keep in mind the goal of every aging-MBB is to maintain a healthy heart and not spend all day running a hamster wheel.

- Subjects with max VO2 scores of 20 to 30 ml/kg/min can comfortably endure 20 to 30 minutes of exercise, 2 to 3 days/week at a BORG scale of 13.

- Subjects with max VO2 scores of 30 to 40 ml/kg/min can comfortably endure 30 to 40 minutes of exercise, 3 to 4 days/week at a BORG scale of 13.

- Subjects with max VO2 scores of 40 to 50 ml/kg/min can comfortably endure 40 to 50 minutes of exercise, 4 to 5 days/week at a BORG scale of 13.

I used this template and created the following aerobic exercise program for Matthew. I suggested he ride a stationary bike for 45 minutes, 4 to 5 days week because his maximal VO2 score was 44.1ml/kg/min. I chose a beginning workload of 180 watts because his BORG scale rating of 13 and his VT matched that workload on the bike.

Initially Matthew asked about increasing the workload to 200 watts because he wanted to burn more calories. The good news is he found it very insightful when I chose to defend my 180-watt workload in terms of calories burned. In his case, the 200-watt effort would only burn an additional 54 calories (1.2 calories more per minute), yet the effort would be significantly more demanding. As expected, he quickly agreed with the 180-watt workload by saying he doubted he could mentally or physically maintain 200 watts for 45 minutes.

I further explained that I had also found the BORG ranking very valuable when subjects are performing steady state cardiovascular exercise. The overwhelming majority of all my test subjects can sustain and maintain workloads that correspond to a 13 to 14 on the BORG scale. Conversely, I have found very few test subjects who are able to train or tolerate steady state efforts at workloads that correspond to a 15 on the BORG scale. More importantly, I have found subjects who started training at a BORG scale rating of 13 to 14 to be more consistent in their adherence to an endurance exercise program.

Today, I still use the same graded exercise testing (GXT) protocol and equipment, because the goals of every cardiovascular exercise program are to improve the heart's ability to deliver oxygenated blood and improve the skeletal muscles' ability to convert food (fat or carbohydrate) into energy. However, I am much more aware that my goal is to design an endurance program that values personal time more than personal performance.

My new question is this: Do the minutes, hours, or days that I take away from someone's life provide a return on things that matter?

Once again, I will use Matthew's GXT data to make my point. In essence, he gave me eighteen hours of his life by agreeing to ride three hours each week (four days/week for forty-five minutes) for six weeks. In return, I needed to show him that cardiovascular exercise was worth his time. To do this, I needed to retest him and show that his new fitness data at 180 watts had improved.

The good news was his retest data showed his 180-watt or 10.2 kcal effort now had a lower heart rate, a lower BORG rating of perceived exertion, his speech was more consistent, and he increased the percentage of fat calories that were being utilized. So he did receive a legitimate return on his personal investment of time, because he showed physiological improvements.

However, my biggest success with him was that his perspective about the amount of time he spent doing aerobic exercise had changed. He now realized his return was not measured by his increased ability to ride a stationary bike. Instead, it meant he could now enjoy all of the other minutes of his day without becoming fatigued. In other words, the return on his investment was best measured in the amount of time and enjoyment when he was off the bike—and that is what really matters.

As an aside, I have always wished that I would find a fitness center with a sign hanging above the exit door that reads, "Go out and enjoy your new level of fitness by spending time doing something that really matters." Sadly, most clubs still believe they exist to provide members a place to come inside and enjoy their life. Yet we know the most important, remarkable, and passionate minutes of life are those that are experienced outside the walls of any fitness center.

The takeaway message is that generic heart rate assumptions are not the best predictor for defining a cardiovascular exercise program's ideal intensity, duration, nor do they predict long-term adherence—which is what really matters.

WHY GENERIC EXERCISE PROGRAMS WON'T WORK—FOR YOU

Let's say a fifty-five-year-old man decides that he needs to start a running program. The first thing he does is buy a high-tech heart rate monitor. He finally decides on a model that continuously measures his heart rate, displays the number on a lightweight wristwatch, and records running time and distance via mile markers with a GPS program. Next, he uses the generic age-predicted heart rate equation and calculates his ideal training heart rate.

With this knowledge, he goes out for a few test runs and fine-tunes his own personalized ideal heart rate. In his case, he finds out that he is able to easily run at a pace that matches a heart rate of 130 bpm. He is so excited about the predictive power of simply using his age to calculate an ideal running heart rate that he buys fifty more heart rate monitors and gives them to fifty other fifty-five-year-old men who are going to run the upcoming marathon. He notices that most of the men are the same size, so he buys everybody matching T-shirts so they can see each other during the marathon.

In return, he shares with them his ideal exercise heart rate calculations for men their age and asks each of them to run their marathon at a pace that would match a heart rate of 135 bpm. He explains that each watch is programmed with an alarm that will chime if their heart rate rises a few beats above the agreed upon 135 bpm, which means they should slow down their running speed. It will also chime if their heart rates drop a few beats below 135 bpm, which means they should run a little faster.

On the morning of the marathon they take a group photo in their matching T-shirts, thank the man for the expensive heart rate monitors, and collectively push the start buttons on their wristwatches at the sound of the starting gun. You'd expect them to run in a pack, right? Pacing at the same distance with similar heart rates.

Wrong. Unfortunately, that is soon to be the last time that this group of same aged men, running the same distance at the same heart rate are anywhere near each other.

The post-race heart rate data clearly showed each man ran at a pace that kept his heart rate very close to 135 bpm. The band of T-shirt-wearing brothers was able to stay in visual contact with each other as they passed through the first few miles, but after they passed the three-mile distance marker, it was clear their marathon finishing time was not determined by their ability to maintain an age-predicted heart rate. Their finishing time—for some the ability to even finish—was determined by their ability to sustain or endure running for 26.2 miles at a heart rate of 135 bpm.

The easiest way to describe the group's marathon finishing times is to put them into three categories: the good, the bad, and the ugly.

The Good: Each man in this category finished the marathon in times varying from 3.5 to 4.5 hours. They never found themselves out of breath or having any difficulty talking. They also perceived the entire course as being only somewhat hard or never higher than a 13 on the BORG scale. Some mentioned they felt held back by being forced to run at a slower pace that matched the 135-bpm heart rate but quickly admitted they really enjoyed the pace, as it allowed them to positively experience the entire marathon. The men with the highest levels of cardiovascular fitness finished ahead of those with lower levels, because they could run faster. The faster runners also burned more calories per minute than the slower runners, but they all burned the same number of total calories because they each performed the same amount of work, and each had similar body weights.

The Bad: While each of these men eventually completed the marathon, their memories weren't particularly joyful. This group's finishing time varied between 5 and 6 hours. Each was more out of breath and had difficulty talking as they neared the 18- to 20-mile markers. Their BORG rating of perceived exertion also changed from being a consistent somewhat hard to an increasing rating of very hard to very, very hard. Sadly, this change became apparent on their faces as each runner approached the final mile markers of what should have been a great accomplishment. Once again, those with the higher levels of fitness finished ahead of the others, yet each of these finishers burned the same numbers of total calories. It just took them much longer to endure the same amount of work.

The Ugly: None of these men were able to finish the marathon. They actually enjoyed the first 3 to 4 miles (30 to 40 minutes) of the marathon and were able to maintain the running pace that matched a heart rate of 135 bpm. However, they all had to slow down their running speed early in the race. Each of these men stated he knew he was in trouble after 5 or 6 miles. Some stated they felt "increasing levels of fatigue" and others "needed to catch their breath." Some were forced to change from running to walking. Eventually, all adopted an alternating combination of walking and jogging that became so interchangeable it was hard to tell if they were moving faster when they were jogging or walking.

Making matters worse, this alternating pattern caused their heart rate watches to continuously chime, because their heart rate had dropped below the programmed 135 bpm. Their frustration continued to mount, and they eventually realized that although their initial 3- to 4-mile effort would be considered a successful workout for a majority of men their age, finishing the marathon would only require them to walk slowly in their expensive running shoes and logo T-shirt while listening to the heart rate monitors chime. Their final thought was that anybody could get up in the morning and start walking for 26.2 miles if they could justify the time.

The takeaway of this example is to consider time when engaging in cardiovascular activity. Do not waste time pretending you are gaining a physiological training effect just because you originally thought it was a good idea. Ironically, we already use "wasting time" as the yes or no variable for a variety of other decisions. My list includes when to leave a sporting event, a boring professional lecture, or a distant relative's wedding reception. My guess is every aging-MBB has uttered both these phrases: "Well, that's six hours of my life that I will never get back," or "That was a complete waste of time." And it was.

CONSIDER YOUR GOAL

One final real-life scenario, a few years ago I was talking with an athletic, lean-looking guy who appeared to be in his midfifties named Adam. Adam shared with me his story of quitting smoking and starting running. He quit because of his daughter's pleading, and he started running because of her personal challenge. Adam had been a heavy smoker for over thirty years and had tried many times to quit, but it was his daughter who finally convinced him to quit.

His first attempts at running were brutal—brutally short in terms of the distance he was able to run and brutally intense in terms of his coughing attacks after those short runs. Adam said, "My life really changed when I realized that I had finally quit smoking and ran two marathons." I congratulated him, and then he asked me a common question. "Do you think I can break the four-hour barrier for my next marathon?" The four-hour barrier has become somewhat of a status symbol for runners who are trying to hold onto their youth.

This question posed a dilemma. I wondered if I should answer this question from an exercise science perspective or from the place of passion and perspective that led me to write this book.

The exercise physiologist in me would have responded by saying, "The great thing about training for improved running performance is that speed is directly tied to your ability to consume oxygen."

I would suggest that we put him on a treadmill and measure his maximal VO2. I would use that data to design an individualized running program that would allow him to run his next marathon under four hours. The program would include monthly retesting to make sure his heart is improving and the mitochondria in his running muscles are improving. He would only need to commit the time, and I could put him on a plan that would take the guesswork out of marathon training.

"The great thing about training for improved running performance is that speed is directly tied to your ability to consume oxygen."

That scenario would be both ethically and scientifically correct. I would be able to improve his marathon time if he would surrender to me his most precious asset—time.

I wrote this book because today my perspective has changed, and I place a much higher value on the exercise variable of time. I no longer feel comfortable assuming it is okay to spend a person's time (days, hours, minutes) without going through the following:

Adam, I said, "I have no problem with your desire to improve your marathon time. However, the thing most runners forget is that distance dictates running speed and running time. For example, today's world-record holder for the mile knows that if he wants to try to set the world record in a longer distance like the 5k (3.1 miles), he would be forced to run at a slower pace than his world-record mile to run the longer distance. This concept translates to other distances as well. It would be the same if he chose to run a 10k (6.2 miles), a half marathon (13.1 miles), or a marathon (26.2 miles). Eventually, each world-record holder discovers that running slower in order to run longer also forces him to set aside more weekly training time, increases his risk of getting injured, and, worse, extends the period of time needed to recover from running slower yet longer.

"I spent time with a five-time Olympic runner who said, 'If you compare competing in the 10k and the marathon, it's much harder to set a world record in the 10k, but it's much harder to recover from running a marathon.' Most importantly, every professional distance runner also realizes the winner of each distance gets the same size gold medal in the Olympics. I want to share that with you, because I want you to rethink your desire to run a marathon under four hours. I want to remind you that your original reason for running was your daughter's wish for you to quit smoking and spend time with her. Her passion for running has enabled the two of you to spend time together. It has also showed you the benefits of having healthy lungs and a strong heart.

"I encourage you to change your focus from running a slow marathon to running a faster 10k. The 10k distance will allow you and your daughter to run side-by-side for the entire race. It will drastically reduce the amount of time you spend practicing to run slow, and you can easily run that distance for the next twenty-five years of your life. If you still want to set performance and age goals, then try finishing every 10k race under 50 minutes through your fifties, under 60 minutes through your sixties, and under 70 minutes through your seventies.

"Finally, I suggest that you choose to enter 10k races that benefit lung cancer. This will allow you and your daughter the flexibility to change your training schedules and to visit different areas of the country. Bottom line for me is you need to remember your daughter was the only person who was able to get you to quit smoking. In essence, she saved your life, which gave you the extra years that most dying cancer patients wish they had. You now have the ability to spend those extra years with her, while simultaneously improving your level of aerobic fitness and encouraging other long-term smokers to quit. Twenty-five years from now you won't know whose heart benefited the most—yours, your daughter's, or the countless number of people you encouraged to quit smoking."

I wanted Adam, like every aging-MBB like us, to do a cost-benefit analysis regarding the amount of time he spends doing aerobic exercise. Stated more bluntly, we all need to view our remaining years of life in terms of the opportunities lost versus the opportunities gained. Having a healthy heart allows us to enjoy spending time doing things that really matter.

For more information about how to measure aerobic fitness levels or the pros and cons of aerobic exercise equipment, visit www.danielzeman.com.

8

OUR LEGACY YEARS, WHAT'S YOURS?

I have always been amazed how the passing of time can shed new light on any historic event. Seems as if those once forgotten or forbidden events can literally become more realistic and meaningful when you put a face on the event. For example, the decision in 2009 to officially recognize the death of the last survivor of the *Titanic* put a human face on that tragic event of 1912.

I realize that every last survivor represented a much larger group of individuals, but it seemed that an era ended with that final death, like the closing of a book. In a similar way, history will eventually place a face on the last survivor of the historic baby boom generation.

What lessons will be learned as our generation sinks beneath the waves? How will we aging male baby boomers be remembered? What were our defining moments?

In the case of the *Titanic*, it is equally important to realize the difference in perspectives between the historians who wrote about the Titanic and the people who survived it. Historians have the ability to sit comfortably and calmly discuss the volumes of crash data plus the clarity of hindsight offered by 20/20 vision of seeing the ancient vessel as it sits on the ocean floor.

Conversely, a survivor on the *Titanic* may have heard screams from fellow travelers or felt cold water rushing down the hallways.

They also faced the possibility that their lives could be over—no long goodbyes, no second chances, just an impending tragic death due to drowning. Those who did survive were forced to spend their remaining years dealing with the physical, financial, and emotional burdens associated with surviving an event that nobody warned them would happen.

I wrote this book because I believe the historic legacy of the longer-living, aging-MBB will be defined by how he chooses to handle the aging process. The key difference between us and those who survived the *Titanic* is that we can plan ahead for the inevitable physical, emotional, and financial burdens that we may have to endure. To me that starts with redefining the word retirement.

Retirement can no longer be viewed or discussed as a single day on the calendar when a looming iceberg tragically hits us. Our ability to retire, like our ability to tolerate the aging process, will depend on the cumulative choices we have made across our lifetime, not on the location of our stateroom aboard a sinking ship.

Every one of us aging-MBBs has been informed that many members of our generation will live past their eighty-fifth birthday.

Every one of us aging-MBBs has been informed that many members of our generation will live past their eighty-fifth birthday. Each has also been told our unhealthy choices will affect our quality of life, our out-of-pocket healthcare costs, and our ability to live independently. In other words, each of us knows that we have the ability to minimize the physical, emotional, and financial burdens that we or someone else will have to pay for our decision to make unhealthy choices.

For those who say they have not been informed, my suggestion is to walk to their old-fashioned mailbox, since it is most likely filled with advertisements on how to plan ahead for their upcoming and expensive retirement.

My biggest motivating factor for writing this book is to enlighten those who believe that all generations are basically the same when it comes to planning ahead for their retirement. They say, "A person is born, lives their life, and then dies." While the simplicity of this belief is true, the reality is that every aging-MBB needs to understand that we were born into the largest generation in history and will live longer than any other generation in history. Most of us will all die within the same relatively short period of time.

YOU CAN SEE THE ICEBERG

Historians have already shown that when the first baby boomers were born in 1946, there were approximately 12 million Americans over the age of sixty-five, of which 600,000 were older than eighty-five. Demographers' predictions for the year 2040 suggest the number of Americans over the age of sixty-five will have increased to 81 million, of which 14 million will be over the age of eighty-five. And for the year 2050, they predict there will be 88.5 million over the age of sixty-five of which 19 million will be over eighty-five.

Let's take a look into the future, to the decade from 2040 to 2050. In 2040, the baby boom generation will range between the ages of seventy-six and ninety-four. In 2050, baby boomers will range between eighty-six and one hundred four years old. Therefore, when the final baby boomer turns eighty-five, he will join a group of 19 million baby boomers who as a generation simply did not die young.

The wake-up call for those 19 million boomers who will reach the age of eighty-five is that each will have had the ability to plan ahead for his retirement. Stated more bluntly, every longer-living, aging-MBB, unlike those who survived the crashing *Titanic*, will not be able to say, "I did not see the iceberg."

Today's updated computer programs will allow historians, actuaries, statisticians, and insurance companies to dissect every piece of data over those final years and provide unprecedented research about the aging process.

These research groups will also be able to demonstrate the long-term aging effects of various factors, such as making unhealthy choices about brain function, memory, use of prescription medications, surgical outcomes, emotional stability, sleep patterns, nutritional status, physical movement patterns, and mental alertness. One of the goals will be to attempt to create a blueprint that will help future generations understand the consequences of making unhealthy choices throughout a lifetime.

A secondary goal of the data analysis will be to show the physical, emotional, and financial costs of every health habit. This will allow researchers to show the cost of compliance versus noncompliance for each habit across the retirement years of every baby boomer. The ability to compare and contrast the medical records, health habits, and health outcomes of such a large group of 19 million people will certainly provide a legitimate cost analysis of the aging process.

As an aside, the use of medical records data is becoming commonplace with many medical conditions. For example, today measurable data show the additional short-term and long-term medical costs for each day of premature birth. These research data were originally designed and used with the hope of improving health outcomes of each newborn baby, but by default, it is also capable of determining the additional daily medical costs of a child being born too early.

Every aging-MBB who has visited an assisted living center would probably agree that living independently for as long as possible will allow us to maintain the highest quality of life. This realization, by default, also means we are choosing to view retirement in financial terms using a cost-savings analysis.

For those who are unfamiliar with the cost of such living arrangements, the typical cost for these facilities in Minnesota in 2017 was $7,000 per month. In other words, every year of delaying a move into assisted living would be an $84,000 cost savings, plus you would be able to maintain a higher quality of life. (Keep in mind that Dr. Atul Gawande stated in his book, *Being Mortal*, that over 80 percent of Americans will end up dying in some type of assisted living center.)

While this should be viewed as a huge win-win for any one of us, historians are only interested in the measurable facts concerning the entire baby boom generation. Their data could easily show Dr. Gawande correct in that 80 percent or (15 million of the 19 million baby boomers) did end up spending their final years in assisted living, which means that each year when all 15 million boomers are paying $84,000 to live in facilities that someone paid somebody $1.26 trillion for this type of housing.

It is not illegal to be unhealthy in America, but it will become very expensive, and someone, some group, or some generation will end up paying the bill for our poor health habits.

In addition, research will also provide mathematical examples of the financial savings if a larger percentage of baby boomers are able to motivate themselves to spend more years living independently. In other words, historians will have the ability to define the daily cost of keeping 19 million baby boomers who are over the age of eighty-five housed, fed, medically safe, and alive. As I previously stated, it is not illegal to be unhealthy in America, but it will become very expensive, and someone, some group, or some generation will end up paying the bill for our poor health habits.

As I mentioned, historians will have access to the billings of every health insurance provider and the medical records of those same populations. They will use the same statistical cost-benefit analysis on every choice that each aging-MBB is able to either adopt or neglect (for example, the annual cost of prescription drugs for a medical condition that is directly tied to a negative personal habit, the cost of ongoing surgeries that is directly tied to a personal habit that he chose to neglect, or the cost of ongoing therapy that is directly tied to a personal habit that he chose to neglect).

The key takeaway is this: We will always have the ability to make personal choices regarding our health habits, but historians will eventually take a very objective perspective and calculate the physical, emotional, and financial costs of the habits we chose to neglect.

The bottom line is to understand that we need to view our retirement as another twenty to twenty-five years of life. We need to view these years as an opportunity to remain productive and socially engaged. We can no longer afford to view retirement as just a few more years before the wheels fall off.

Forrest Gump asked his dying mother, "What is my destiny, Mama?" I will instead end the book by asking you, "What is your legacy?"

My request is based on my belief that a person's destiny is something he achieves prior to his retirement, but his legacy is something that encompasses his entire lifetime. More importantly, a person's legacy will be how his friends and family remember him.

The following examples of notable men should help explain the difference between a destiny and a legacy.

- Bob Dylan was destined to become a singer/songwriter.

- Bill Gates was destined to become a computer entrepreneur.

- Francis Collins was destined to become a physician.

It is fair to say that each achieved his destiny, but historians will make sure to include their legacies.

- Bob Dylan went on to become a Nobel Prize winner in literature and continues to tour the world sharing his poetic message.

- Bill Gates went on to become world-renowned for his work in improving the health of vulnerable people in developing countries.

- Francis Collins went on to become known for his work involving the human genome project and is currently the director of the National Institutes of Health.

In essence, each of these men understands that retirement is not an age-driven line in the sand. Instead, each has decided to spend time expanding or adding new opportunities to what can only be described as another chapter to his life.

I realize that many of us aging male baby boomers will not be able to continue our previous occupation due to the intense demands of those jobs. Some may be legally required to retire at an age-driven line in the sand, but that does not mean you have no other marketable qualities or worthy attributes.

Find satisfaction that you are destined to become an expert in your field—but your legacy will be defined by how you choose to spend the remainder of your life after your occupational career is over.

It is also safe to say that how you spend those extra years, months, days, and precious minutes will show future generations whether the male baby boomer chose to redefine the word retirement because you cared about your legacy.

ARE YOU READY TO PLAY?

In 1982, the NBA created the Sixth Man of the Year Award after they realized they had players who placed a high value on number of minutes on the court. Each of these players understood that getting on the court and playing the game was their only goal. These players were not motivated by the desire to be recognized during the pregame introduction, obtain the biggest contract, or have the elite name recognition. The only thing each understood was that someday he would turn in his jersey and never play basketball again. But until that day, his favorite words were, "Put me in, coach, I'm ready to play today!"

Additionally, if you asked other NBA players about those players who won the Sixth Man of the Year Award, they would say, "When he came on the court, he literally changed the mood of the game," or "He just made everybody want to play better," or "You could tell he just loved and cherished those minutes." Today the Sixth Man of the Year Award has an impressive list of talented players, most of whom have become household names.

What does this award mean for you? One day we'll each turn in our playing jerseys. And wouldn't it be great if each of us received those types of accolades from friends, family, or people who only saw us from afar? You were always ready to play.

For those who are not motivated by sports analogies, let me suggest another option. In the bible, Psalm 128 infers that a blessed man is one who will live long enough to see his children's children. In essence, over two thousand years ago, a man would be considered blessed to have good health, as it would allow him to live long enough to experience the joys of being a grandparent.

While I still find value in that scripture passage, I never asked my grandparents if they ever felt blessed by living long enough to see me. In fact, I still believe that I was blessed to be able to spend time with them. My grandfather taught me about fishing, tractors, crops, and how to stay out of trouble. My grandmother taught me about folding clothes, cooking, religion, and how to treat girls.

I also never thought of my grandparents as being healthy or unhealthy. All I remember is they remained physically active, mentally engaged, and financially stable enough to live independently for all but a few days of their lives. Most importantly, many other baby boomers and I view the legacy of grandparents through those same childhood eyes and are still able to smile when looking at those old black-and-white photographs.

To me, every photograph or memory of my aging grandparents reminds me of the importance they placed on their final years, months, days, and minutes on earth. Clearly, they knew life had a beginning and an end, but they continued to find enjoyment in the minutes they had together.

In light of Psalm 128, ask yourself two simple questions: Will I consider it a blessing to live long enough to see not only my children's children but the children of my children's children? And will my grandchildren and great grandchildren view my legacy in the same positive fashion that I view my grandparents' legacy?

Looking back, I would say my grandparents had three characteristics that today's aging-MBB could use as a blueprint on how to battle the aging process. The first was their attitudes and personalities. The second was their intrinsic drive to remain physically active and mentally engaged. The third was their desire to live together in a house that celebrated their past and always smelled like a small-town bakery.

With regard to your attitude and personality: I am convinced your personality is something that you are born with, but your attitude is an everyday decision. This means the generational comparison is really about how we can choose to maintain a positive attitude. The biggest controllable variable that will help us with this decision every morning to have a positive attitude is our overall health status.

I suggest you begin implementing my twelve habits because nobody wants to be around an aging old man with a negative attitude. Certainly, everyone has already met this man and has walked away saying, "Wow that is one crabby, angry, grumpy old man, and I hope I never have to see him again!"

With regard to your intrinsic drive: I believe each generation finds or creates its own intrinsic drive. My grandparents' drive came from surviving the Depression, the dust bowl, and the challenging living conditions of the 1920s and 1930s on the family farm. Their daily decision to remain physically active and mentally engaged became as habitual as tying their shoes.

In a similar fashion, our generation found our intrinsic drive within the political and social change of the 1960s and 1970s. Songs documented us as being a generation with a new vision. We believed in bridging the economic gap between the haves and have-nots, and most importantly we wanted a nation of equal rights and equal responsibilities for everyone. The passion to improve the country became an intrinsic driving force.

My suggestion for those of us who have lost our intrinsic drive is to begin a weekly plan that incorporates the types of activities that I have discussed in this book. You will begin to notice an immediate improvement in your physical capabilities and mental alertness. Your family, friends, children, and grandchildren will find enjoyment in your renewed desire to go for a walk, hike, or bike ride with them or attend their events.

The desire to remain mentally engaged is the other way you can show your spouse, family, children, and grandchildren that you care about them. To this day, I still don't know if my grandfather's story about how he had to walk five miles to the one-room schoolhouse in the snow without any shoes was fact or fiction, but it really doesn't matter. The only thing that matters is that I remember him as a man who remained mentally engaged and fun to be around.

With regard to your desire to remain living in your home: I admired my grandparents' generation's passionate desire to live in their home, but the fact is that the baby boom generation will live much longer lives and will be forced to deal with the nonstop physical decline that is associated with the aging process. Eventually, we will begin to recognize the difference between our emotional desires and our physical abilities.

The best example of having the desire but not the ability is driving an automobile. Most boomers have already noticed their ability to drive is being influenced by a decrease in night vision, hearing loss, upper body mobility, or frustration found in dealing with the faster speeds of other drivers. These scenarios do not change your desire to drive, but they provide clear examples of how the aging process can deteriorate your ability to safely drive.

I have great news. The easy solution that will save money is for every aging-MBB to simply sell his car, quit paying for auto insurance and expensive repairs, and switch to using a variety of door-to-door shuttle services such as Uber and Lyft. This creates an easy win-win solution. For those who can't imagine selling their car, there is also an easy lose-lose solution. There will be a day when your failure to prepare for the loss of ability, agility, and coordination will result in your inability to pass the driving-under-the-influence test. You will fail not because you are drunk but under the influence of aging. The cost of the ticket and the embarrassment will definitely be a lose-lose scenario.

Unfortunately, the desire to continue to live in your home and still maintain the physical ability to live in your home does not have a simple solution. Most baby boomers have already noticed a decrease in their ability to climb steps, do yardwork, or perform basic home maintenance. Most have already tried downsizing or moving to single-floor maintenance-free villas and condos. Others have tried removing the physical demands inside their house by purchasing equipment or furniture that lifts and lowers their body. These products do reduce the work-loads, but they also increase the rate of muscle atrophy caused by inactivity and the aging process.

I am not opposed to household products that are marketed under the safety slogan of "I have fallen and I can't get up," but the slogan should be updated for those sedentary sofa-flopping male boomers to say, "I have fallen and I forgot how to get up."

View your ability to live independently as a benchmark or cornerstone for your retirement years. I believe the longer-living male baby boomer will not be defined by his philosophical desires but by his ability to continually motivate himself to remain physically, mentally, and emotionally able to live in his home throughout his lifetime.

A TITANIC WAVE IS COMING

The next twenty-five to thirty years will be a time of great change in America. The simple fact is nobody—government, churches, charities, housing, transportation, and certainly not healthcare—planned for the consequences caused by the drastic rise in life expectancy in America. The wake-up call for every aging-MBB is to realize his retirement years may coincide with political finger pointing, changes in federal tax laws and Medicare, and healthcare reform.

Similar to the *Titanic's* last survivor, the media will seek to put a face on the last surviving boomer and then close the book on our generation. Historians will begin to calculate the cost that we—the largest and longest-living generation—had on such things as the environment and healthcare. Our children will begin to discuss the private battles they witnessed as to how each Dad dealt with the aging process and when each man chose to quit fighting for the extra years, days, and minutes of his life.

I am convinced that the legacy of the aging-MBB will be defined by how he eventually chooses to deal with the last two to three decades of his life—his retirement years!

There really are only two possible options.

We can choose to view retirement as a time to become lethargic, financially irresponsible, socially unengaged, and physically inactive to the point where we become unable to get up off the coach and volunteer at the plethora of charities we created. We will then be viewed as the greatest generational irony in modern history. In essence, we will be remembered as a generation of men who began preaching a message of social change and personal responsibility but ended up asking for a disproportionate amount of financial assistance caused by our poor choices. Our dying words will be, "I didn't see the iceberg."

We can choose to view retirement as a time to become more passionate and appreciative of the bonus gift of a longer life.

Or we can choose to view retirement as a time to become more passionate and appreciative of the bonus gift of a longer life. We will redefine the aging process and, more importantly, become the new role model for how Americans view the elderly. In essence, we can be remembered as a generation of men who understand we have been given the gift of a longer life and the freedom to make personal choices, and we choose to spend our bonus years staying physically active, mentally engaged, and living independently.

My hope is you have found a renewed motivation to leave the legacy that initially defined the baby boom generation, as well as appreciate the urgency of your decision to choose to age with dignity.

ACKNOWLEDGMENTS

I started writing this book in the year 2000. I admit there are some people whose names I will forget to mention and some whom I never knew the role they played in my personal or professional development.

Knowing that, let me start by acknowledging editor Melissa Johnson who made my words become a story. You are gifted and skilled beyond words that I could ever express.

To the team at Concierge Marketing Publishing Services, you truly heard my vision and created a package that is a remarkable extension of my words. Your care and passion to help me share my life's work are evident in everything you do.

As for the rest on my list:

Dr. Herb Schoening was the first to believe in my professional abilities. I would like to state how nervous I became many years later when I was giving a speech and recognized that you were sitting in the front row.

Other physicians include the original Minneapolis Sports Medicine Center group: Dr. David Fischer, Dr. Alan Markman, Dr. John Boyd, and Dr. John Stuebs. Thank you for the respect you have always shown me as it gave me the confidence to write this book. Also, Dr. Brett Oden for sharing his personal story that years of intense ultra-endurance training does produce victories, but the cost of lost lean body mass and personal time outweighs the potential for long-term health benefits.

Acknowledging the athletes in my life is a must because they provided me a much broader perspective on the aging process. Three of them in particular need formal recognition. Greg LeMond. We met doing VO2 testing, but I thank you for including me on every road, path, or trail that we have traveled off the bike. Mark Madsen. We met through the Timberwolves, but I thank you for everything we have done off the basketball court. Team Heart (Dan Dunn, Phil Murray, Tom Pettus, Bob Mackie). We met trying to improve your chances of riding a bike from Oregon to Florida in seven days. Thank you for allowing me to help raise money for the hearts of an unknown number of children.

Acknowledging the musicians in my life is a must because sitting on the stages of their shows convinced me that I needed to strike a familiar chord with my audience if I were to create long-term adherence. Thank you, Paul English, Mickey Raphael, John Selman, Scott Joss, Frank Mull, Baron Tabura, Mike Ramos, Duane Allen, Joe Bonsall, Darrick Kinslow, Jimmy Burton, and Lisa Kristofferson for inviting me to hang backstage during the shows.

Next, an alphabetical list of individuals who convinced me that my book was worth reading and without them I would not have written it. Joe Bonsall, an author who shares my belief that the baby boomers' gift of "freedom of choice" was paid for by those buried in places like Arlington Cemetery. Tom Branham, a dentist with great teeth and a better ear for good music. Sean Couillard, who reps the most comfortable treadmill but always had time to sit on a bad chair and have a good cup of coffee. Andre Deloya, the single greatest "hands-on" physical therapist I have ever met. Daniel De Vise, a successful author who shares my belief in the value of maintaining male friendships. Gregg Farnam, an athletic trainer who has been one of my biggest supporters. Dave Fischer, an orthopedic surgeon whose words of encouragement provided me the closure I needed to finish my book. Tom Gullickson, a tennis hall of famer who lost his twin but never quit the game of life. Dean Hovey, a Stanford graduate with insight, intelligence, and integrity. Bruce Johnson, a clinical researcher whose foundation is on solid ground. Scott

Joss, a prolific reader but most nights preferred the lyrics to "Sing me back home before I die." Lisa Kristofferson, a person who remembers that memories are constantly being created in the aging brain. Greg Lappin, a guy who defines the word friend. Paul Magers, a very talented and nationally recognized TV anchor who decided to choose a healthier life. Mike Max, for allowing me to chat on his airwaves. Bill McGuire, an individual for whom I have the utmost respect. Kevin McHale, an NBA hall of famer who, win or lose, still values his playing minutes. Mickey Raphael, a harmonica player who showed me the power of inhaling and exhaling for those you love. Arnold Schwarzenegger, an icon who said "write your book," shared his reasons why and then promised when it is finished, "I will be back". Bill Schiebler, a Vietnam veteran with a bronze star and a kind heart. Scott Sechrest, a fit guy with whom I share the same vison on how to upgrade the fitness business. Neal Sher, an ophthalmologist who quickly saw the vision for my book by looking through the eyes of his aging parents. And to John Ullrich, a software legend born in Wisconsin with dreams of ASPEN, but who remained a constant companion in my life.

My final acknowledgments are to my family: my older and younger brothers, Steve and Mike, for literally being two powerful bookends to my life's content. My wife, Marilyn, who reminds me every day that males and females are genetically different, but together they can create a book that is worth reading and a life that is worth living.

ABOUT THE AUTHOR

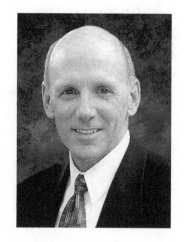

Dan Zeman is an exercise physiologist with extensive experience in health, fitness, and sports medicine. He has designed exercise programs for professional athletes in the National Hockey League, National Football League including the Minnesota Vikings, National Basketball Association including the Minnesota Timberwolves and three-time Tour de France winner, cyclist Greg LeMond.

But Zeman's real passion is working with aging Americans, and this book is the result of a three-decade career working with individuals of all ages and fitness levels. He holds a master's degree in exercise physiology from the University of North Texas.

He began working in a clinical setting with heart attack survivors and people with diabetes.

During his career, he has conducted an array of research involving the aerobic capacities of wheelchair athletes, a comparison study of today's child to different types of free play and a seven-year longitudinal study comparing the fitness levels of AAU girls' basketball players.

Zeman has consulted with corporations that manufacture metabolic testing equipment, body fat measuring devices, and traditional exercise equipment. He also provides expertise for computer software firms that design health and fitness packages for hospitals, fitness centers, and corporate wellness centers.

He's the go-to expert for today's cutting-edge technology companies that design web-driven medical and fitness-related exercise products.

He has appeared on a variety of television and radio programs, has been featured in magazine and newspaper articles, and continues to create content for his www.danielzeman.com website including Podcast under the title of "A 46-64 Perspective".

He and his wife, Marilyn, live in Scottsdale, Arizona.

CPSIA information can be obtained
at www.ICGtesting.com
Printed in the USA
LVHW111402170421
684796LV00032B/563

9 780960 061921